Healing Back
and
Joint Injuries

A Proven Approach *to*
Ending Chronic Pain *and*
Avoiding Unnecessary Surgery

JOSEPH VALDEZ, MD, MS

WITH CONTRIBUTIONS BY MIGUEL PAPPOLLA, MD

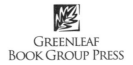

GREENLEAF
BOOK GROUP PRESS

This book is intended as a reference volume only, not as a medical manual. The information given here is designed to help you make informed decisions about your health. It is not intended as a substitute for any treatment that may have been prescribed by your doctor. If you suspect that you have a medical problem, you should seek appropriate medical help.

Published by Greenleaf Book Group Press
Austin, Texas
www.greenleafbookgroup.com

Distributed by Greenleaf Book Group LLC

For ordering information or special discounts for bulk purchases, please contact Greenleaf Book Group LLC at PO Box 91869, Austin, TX 78709, 512.891.6100.

Design and composition by Greenleaf Book Group LLC
Illustrations by Brad Albright
Cover design by Greenleaf Book Group LLC

Cataloging-in-Publication data
(Prepared by the Donohue Group, Inc.)

Valdez, Joseph.
   Healing back and joint injuries : a proven approach to ending chronic pain
and avoiding unnecessary surgery / Joseph Valdez with Miguel Pappolla. – 1st ed.

   p. : ill. ; cm.

   Includes bibliographical references and index.
   ISBN: 978-1-929774-79-1

1. Chronic pain—Treatment—Popular works. 2. Chronic pain—Alternative treatment. 3. Back—Wounds and injuries—Treatment—Popular works. 4. Joints—Wounds and injuries—Treatment—Popular works. I. Pappolla, Miguel. II. Title.

RB127 .V25 2009
616/.0472   2009928416

 Part of the Tree Neutral™ program, which offsets the number of trees consumed in the production and printing of this book by taking proactive steps, such as planting trees in direct proportion to the number of trees used: www.treeneutral.com

Printed in the United States of America on acid-free paper

09 10 11 12 13 14   10 9 8 7 6 5 4 3 2 1

First Edition

Contents

Introduction

Freddie was my two oldest boys' soccer coach. When he arrived at the field, he would immediately lie down and conduct practice from this position. After watching him direct the players this way several weeks in a row, my wife asked Freddie's wife what was wrong. It was no surprise to learn that Freddie was in severe discomfort. His wife explained that while doing leg lifts one day, he had experienced a sharp pain in his lower back that had remained ever since. In fact, because of the constant irritation, Freddie was having difficulty performing his job as a police officer, let alone his side duties as a soccer coach. He had seen his regular physician and been referred to an orthopedist, who had him undergo a magnetic resonance imaging test (MRI). While looking at the MRI results, and before conducting a physical examination, the orthopedist recommended surgery. Freddie and his wife wanted to know whether this was his only option.

Barbara was even worse off than the soccer coach. She was told she would have to live the rest of her life in suffering, the type that could never be fully controlled or eased. When I first met her, she was a sad and tired fifty-four-year-old. She had hurt her back some years before and had been living with severe, chronic pain. After not improving with the usual conservative treatments, Barbara underwent back surgery, with excellent initial results. In fact, she had no significant back problems for years. But her lower back pain eventually returned. This time, the debilitating pain was accompanied by discomfort in the right buttock, so much so that sitting provoked sharp twinges that radiated down her right leg. Barbara had always enjoyed gardening, but planting and weeding caused her too much discomfort. Repetitive bending and pulling wasn't possible anymore. By the time I met her, the pain had become constant and severe despite narcotic medications and steroid injections. At times, Barbara was even unable to get out of bed. At other times, she could not stay in bed. It had become impossible to find a comfortable position to relieve the agony for more than a few fleeting moments.

Is your story anything like Freddie's or Barbara's? If so, you definitely need this book. Is the problem you face much less severe than theirs? If so, you also definitely need this book. Why? Because, let's face it, getting injured is a part of life—especially if you lead an active, dynamic life. How we deal with the injuries we experience, even the minor ones, can determine the quality of our lives from that point forward. Nobody wants to suffer a minor injury and then make a bad treatment decision that leads to chronic pain. And we shouldn't have to.

WHY YOU NEED THIS BOOK

1. **You have a back or joint soft tissue injury**—and possibly a chronic injury—and you're trying to understand what has happened in your body and how to treat it effectively and permanently.
2. **You suffer from chronic joint or back pain** and you're seeking relief.
3. **You've been told you need surgery to correct a back or joint injury**, but you want to understand what your options are first.
4. **You are trying to help a loved one** who is facing one of these problems.

After sixteen years of treating injuries and chronic pain of all kinds, I can say with certainty that when we make informed choices about how to manage our health and the injuries that inevitably occur, we can lead active, pain-free lives. I wrote this book because I have seen too many people make the wrong decisions about how to treat their physical ailments, too many people live with unnecessary discomfort, and too many people undergo unnecessary surgery with negative outcomes — physical, emotional, and even financial. What causes this? And why is it so common? The simple answer to both of those questions is this: The current surgical and medical protocols often lead to misdiagnosis of one of the most common types of injury — soft tissue — and mistreatment of the most common cause of pain — connective tissue injuries.

Soft tissue injuries most commonly involve tendons, ligaments, and muscles — sometimes all three. While there are other types of soft tissue in our bodies, muscular and connective tissues are those that are usually injured and are therefore the primary topic of this book. A doctor may have told you that you have a strain, sprain, repetitive stress injury, or subluxation. These are all soft tissue injuries.

SOFT TISSUE INJURIES ARE MORE COMMON THAN YOU MIGHT THINK

- Sprains and strains are one of the top three types of injury that result in emergency room visits (the others are open wounds and contusions).
- From 2002 to 2004, more than 5.5 million people visited emergency rooms *each year* for sprains and strains.
- More than 50,000 people, on average, were hospitalized each year for sprains and strains in 2002 to 2004.
- Almost 44 percent of injuries occurred in or around the home (National Center for Health Statistics, 2006).

The most important thing to understand when facing a soft tissue injury is that it can easily be worsened. Delays in treatment or general mistreatment of the injury are the two primary ways it can become chronic pain. And unfortunately, delays and mistreatment happen too often. One reason why is that diagnosing and treating soft tissue injuries is difficult and often involve ruling out other types of injuries, usually by having the patient undergo a variety of tests. Treatment is prescribed for a condition that wasn't ruled out rather than for a firm diagnosis of what is actually wrong. Patients wait and wait until a doctor finally tells them he or she thinks they have a soft tissue injury because nothing else seems to be wrong. During that waiting period, a hurt knee is still bending, a weakened ankle is still bearing weight, and strained back muscles are still being used on a daily basis. All the while, the injury is worsening.

I saw too many people suffering with these types of injuries and receiving poor advice about how to manage them, so I became devoted to treating them as part of my family practice. And because my passion for helping them led me to research the best solution, I found prolotherapy. Even though you may not have heard of prolotherapy before now, don't interpret that to mean it isn't a viable, respected form of treatment. Hundreds of physicians practice prolotherapy. Numerous studies have been conducted—with more being done every day—that have proven its effectiveness. In fact, the journal *Practical Pain Management* introduced a prolotherapy department in 2007, and the Mayo Clinic, one of the nation's most respected medical establishments, uses prolotherapy to treat its patients' low back pain.

In the sixteen years I have treated people's joint and back pain with prolotherapy, I have seen hundreds of people achieve amazing results. I have seen patients who refused surgery—even though a surgeon had told them it was "the only option"—make complete recoveries and resume working and maintaining an active or even strenuous lifestyle. I have seen patients overcome years of chronic pain and return to the lives they knew before the injury. And I have seen patients quickly and fully heal after injuries that could have left them disabled for life.

What Is Prolotherapy?

You're probably wondering, what exactly is prolotherapy? Prolotherapy is short for proliferative therapy, also known as reconstructive therapy or a type of regenerative injection therapy. It is a nonsurgical treatment that works by strengthening worn ligaments and tendons that no longer support their skeletal structures properly, either because they've been injured or because they've been misused, which will lead to injury over time. Prolotherapy involves a series of injections of nonpharmacological solutions (often dextrose, a sugar solution) that restore cartilage and strengthen ligaments and tendons. The solutions do this by irritating the tissues in the area, stimulating the body's natural response to injury, and causing the body to begin the natural steps toward healing.

Our bodies typically repair connective tissue through inflammation, which increases blood flow and the production of growth factors in an injured area to promote healing. But cartilage, tendons, and ligaments have poor blood supplies. Consequently, they often do not heal completely after an injury, even though the body sends more blood to injured areas just for this purpose. Incomplete healing leads to pain because the structures can no longer adequately hold up their end of the bargain—keeping bones aligned and muscles functioning properly.

> The more you become injured and the longer your injuries go untreated, the weaker and more stretched your ligaments become.

The more you become injured and the longer your injuries go untreated, the weaker and more stretched your ligaments and tendons become. This results in a poor support system and discomfort. The ligaments and tendons of knees, elbows, wrists, shoulders, and other major joints are subject to wear and tear from overuse and injury. Think of a ligament as a rubber band; now, imagine one that is stretched out, thin—in other words, a useless item. But if you could restore its thickness and strength, your ligament could once again hold up the structures it was designed to support, protecting you from unnecessary injury and pain.

That's what prolotherapy does: The injections restore weakened ligaments and tendons because they cause inflammation in areas that don't typically get a sufficient blood supply to heal completely on their own. Prolotherapy is most effective when it is used in combination with other therapies, such as physical therapy, that help relieve associated physiological problems. But using those therapies without addressing the injured, weak connective tissues will only result in repeated injury and recurrent pain.

Should You Consider Prolotherapy?

Prolotherapy can be used to treat a wide range of problems. It has been found to be most effective in treating connective tissue injuries of the knee, hip, wrist, shoulder, and lower back. But I have also had much success using it to treat a host of other physical ailments, including whiplash injuries, weakened ankles, and others.

Prolotherapy does have its drawbacks. It involves multiple injections, which makes some patients uncomfortable. It may not be covered by your insurance plan. It can cause temporary pain at the injection site. And it is not appropriate for every type of soft tissue injury. However, prolotherapy may be the very best treatment for you.

WHEN SHOULD YOU CONSIDER PROLOTHERAPY?

If you answer yes to any of the following questions, prolotherapy may be the right choice for you (Faber, 2007):

- Do you take anti-inflammatory drugs, such as aspirin, naproxen, or ibuprofen, to manage chronic pain?
- Do your painful joints make grinding, popping, clicking, or snapping sounds?
- Do you have joint stiffness, aching, and inflammation in or around your joints?
- Have you had synovitis, tendinitis, or another musculoskeletal problem?
- Do you use a brace, splint, or supportive strapping for an uncomfortable body part?

- Have you experienced only temporary relief from chiropractic adjustments, osteopathic manipulation, massage, myofascial release, acupressure, or other forms of bodywork?
- Does your joint discomfort lessen when at rest and worsen after exercise (except swimming and bicycling)?
- Have you undergone surgery to repair or correct tendons, ligaments, carpal tunnel syndrome, herniated discs, chronic joint dislocation, or other related conditions, but you still experience pain?
- Do you sleep poorly and wake up in the middle of the night or in the morning in pain?
- Do you have difficulty getting out of a chair, walking down stairs, or turning over in bed?

When you are looking for a remedy for your injury and a solution to your discomfort, consider prolotherapy along with all of your other treatment options. If you have been injured in the past and the basic medical treatments haven't helped, consider prolotherapy treatment. If you have recently suffered an injury and are seeking a different solution for your pain, consider prolotherapy treatment right away. Don't live with chronic pain for years, and don't risk further injuring yourself. Take a lesson from Freddie and Barbara.

Needless to say, Freddie wanted to avoid surgery, but he hadn't been presented with any other options. He was ready to agree to surgery until my wife, seeing him lying on the soccer field sidelines, suggested he come see me. At his first visit, Freddie was obviously in severe discomfort and unable to walk normally. He complained of severe pain radiating down his right leg as well as intense discomfort in his lower back. My examination revealed that his pain was not consistent with that which results from a herniated disc, so I explained prolotherapy to Freddie. He was very eager to start the treatment, but because he had been told that his MRI revealed a herniated disc, we postponed his first injection until after I reviewed his MRI. I received a copy of the MRI and consulted with a radiologist, expecting the diagnosis to be either wrong or exaggerated, but the radiologist pointed out a huge herniated disc. My heart sank: Freddie would need surgery.

At his follow-up visit, I told Freddie that the MRI did indeed show a large herniated disc and, in light of his severe pain, I recommended surgery. Freddie, however, was unmoved. He insisted I try prolotherapy first. I explained to Freddie that to delay surgery could result in permanent nerve damage from the herniated disc, which I thought must have been impinging on a nerve, considering his MRI results. Freddie held his ground. He had already suffered for several months, and he resolved to wait a few more weeks in hopes of experiencing successful results with prolotherapy. After all, he said, what did he have to lose?

Reluctantly, I agreed to one or two treatments. If they were unsuccessful, Freddie agreed to undergo the surgery. Incredibly, Freddie was markedly better after just two treatments, and his pain totally resolved with a few more. The herniated disc seen on the MRI remains, but his discomfort is gone. Thus, in his case, it appeared that the herniated disc was not the cause of his pain and that the disc wasn't interfering with the nerves in his spine. Surgery wasn't necessary. What I didn't know then, but was to discover later, was that many people — "normal," pain-free people — have MRIs that show they have a herniated disc, but they never experience any symptoms.

When Barbara came to see me, she had been suffering for three years. Based on Barbara's history and her physical, I concluded that her pain had actually begun with her back surgery, years prior to the return of the pain. Despite being both necessary and successful at the time of surgery, the laminectomy (removal of bone tissue from vertebrae) laid the foundation for her present condition. It had, in essence, weakened her spine. Ordinarily, the body's weight is distributed equally down the pelvis and into the legs. The surgery resulted in an inappropriate amount of weight being shifted to Barbara's right side. This extra stress over time began to affect her right iliolumbar ligaments and her right sacroiliac (SI) joint. After her back surgery, Barbara avoided regular exercise for fear of reinjuring herself. Her decreased activity, plus the onset of menopause, resulted in weight gain that added to the pressure on her joints. Her chronic pain, menopause, and stress led to lack of sleep and general fatigue.

The first order of the day was to treat her severe discomfort. Barbara began to receive prolotherapy to the ligament that connects her lower spine to her pelvis (the iliolumbar ligament) and to the ligaments of her right SI joint (the joint between the base of the spine, the sacrum, and the iliac crest of the pelvis). Almost immediately, the pain became much less severe, and intermittent rather than constant. After three treatments, Barbara began to feel that prolotherapy was helping. Before long, she was able to tolerate more activity. After six treatments, Barbara began to do simple household chores, such as mopping and sweeping. She was able to bend over to pick things up without thinking about the agony her actions might provoke. Sitting and walking were becoming much more comfortable. Her sleep improved. After fourteen treatments her back pain and the pain that had radiated down her right leg were gone. She even returned, though slowly and carefully, to her favorite hobby of gardening. Her life was now active and flourishing again. Barbara continued to be treated for other health issues related to her age and weight, but her outlook was on the upswing.

> To help you make a smart, informed decision about treating an injury, managing chronic pain, or undergoing surgery, I will educate you about your options.

What This Book Offers You

To help you make a smart, informed decision about treating an injury, managing chronic pain, or undergoing surgery, I will educate you about your options. In the pages of this book, I explain

- What is happening in your body—how you've injured yourself or why you're experiencing discomfort,
- What the typical treatment regimen might be,
- The various alternatives that should be considered, and

- How prolotherapy should fit into your overall plan for treatment if you want long-term healing and relief of pain.

My hope is that after reading *Healing Back and Joint Injuries*, you will be able to avoid making the kinds of mistakes I see many patients—and doctors—make. This book is written for all those patients whose doctors maintain that their chronic pain is in their head. This book is written for all those patients in mild to severe pain who are told they must have surgery after basic efforts to remedy the problem have failed. This book is written for people who want to understand what's happening in their body and how to fix the real problems.

Are you tired of being in agony? Are you saddened to see your friend or family member suffer with chronic back or joint injury? Are you ready to take a step toward being healthy? Would you like to be able to return to the life you knew before a step or a bend or a stretch became too painful to bear?

Be proactive about your health! If you think prolotherapy might help you, read on.

Chapter 1

What It Means to Be Injured

Andres is a sixty-five-year-old man who was afflicted with polio as a young boy. He walks with a noticeable limp because the disease weakened his right leg. As a result of this weakness, his left leg has had to support a disproportionate amount of his weight when he walks. Over time, as you might expect, this has led to considerable pain. Several years before I met Andres, he had consulted a number of specialists for the moderately severe pain in his left leg. When he came to see me, however, it was not for help treating his chronic pain; he was simply looking for a general family physician. By the time Andres and I met, he had undergone several MRIs, had received epidural steroid injections, was taking methadone and another medication for nerve pain, and had a nerve stimulator implanted in his back. Despite all that, he was still miserable from the pain. Andres had been more debilitated by his treatment, specifically the narcotics, than he had been by his polio.

You might not think of Andres as having a soft tissue injury. In fact, you probably think of him as disabled in some way. But Andres was injured. His injury was a result of the improper functioning of his right leg, but it was an injury nonetheless.

Why Being Injured Is a Better Outlook

Many people, particularly those who have been suffering with certain afflictions for some time, don't think of their problems as injuries. They say, rather, that they suffer from chronic pain or that they are disabled. The problem with thinking in those terms is that it leaves no room to hope for any better quality of life. If you have chronic pain, more than likely you believe — because you've been told to — that your only option is drug management. Your pain will never go away, and likely won't even lessen. You're relegated to a life of pain and medications, such as opioids (also called narcotics), that will likely become less effective over time. How does one cope with that outlook? If you think of yourself as disabled, more than likely you believe that you will never be able to do the things you once enjoyed in life or never be fully active again. You fear that you will never have the full, normal, healthy use of your body. Again, how does one cope with that outlook?

What if, instead, you started to think of yourself as injured? Some of you reading this book think about your current situation that way already because you have recently injured yourself. Maybe you're an athlete who has twisted your ankle or overextended your knee. Maybe you have a physical job and injured your back lifting a load that was just a bit too heavy. But even if your pain wasn't caused by a single precipitating event, I propose that you should think of your problem as an injury.

Why? For two positive reasons: (1) Injuries can heal, and (2) injuries are temporary — they can be treated and you can recover. Now isn't that a much better outlook than life in pain or life without hope of returning to your normal activities?

I'm not saying that every physical problem can be treated as an injury or can be remedied. But what I am saying is that we should always seek ways to heal our bodies, not just treat the symptoms that we experience as a result of our injuries. If you go to the root, to the place where the injury originates, and you treat that place and heal that spot, the symptoms will disappear, along with any other residual effects on your body.

Let's look at Andres again. When I examined Andres, he experienced significant pain along the muscle tendons in his left lower leg when I applied pressure there. I believed that those tendons had been overly stressed—injured—as a result of the malfunction of his right leg, so I recommended we try prolotherapy, and Andres agreed to give it a literal shot. A few months later, after several courses of prolotherapy, cortisone, and trigger point injections in the area of pain, Andres was off methadone and his other nerve medications, and his spinal nerve stimulator had been removed. He continues to have mild pain, for which he takes Tylenol and an occasional mild narcotic to help him sleep through the night. But overall, Andres's life has been substantially improved by the use of prolotherapy because the effect of repeated stress to the joints in his left leg has been treated directly. Andres can now go shopping or walk to the school fair, becoming part of the family again. His ligaments and tendons are stronger and support his frame better. He had an injury, and it has been healed. He will likely continue to injure the tendons in his left leg because of the persistent malfunction of his right leg, but prolotherapy can continue to heal that, and now he has an outlook that involves healing and recovery.

> Injuries are temporary—they can be treated and you can recover.

To help you change your outlook and understand what's happening in your body, I'm going to explain the different types of connective tissue injuries we experience. If you are seeing a doctor for a specific injury, you should have received a thorough explanation of what has gone wrong in a given joint or in your back. I invite you to skip around in this chapter and read the sections that are most relevant to your situation. I'm going to begin by giving you a basic anatomy lesson on joints and the back.

Joint Anatomy 101

Your joints are made up of multiple types of tissues that work together to support your frame and allow you to move freely. Most of the joints we'll be discussing in this book are called synovial joints. These are the joints that offer the most range of movement, and consequently, they are the least stable and the most prone to injury. Synovial joints are formed where two or more bones meet but are not directly joined to each other, for example, the shoulder, elbow, wrist, hip, knee, and ankle joints. The primary elements that make up these joints are cartilage, synovial tissue, ligaments, and bones. And these joints wouldn't be able to operate (allow us to move) if our muscles weren't connected to our bones through tendons, which will be discussed after the key joint structures. It is the soft tissues in and around joints that prolotherapy is designed to treat.

Cartilage

There are different types of cartilage in the human body. The cartilage in joints is a type of hyaline cartilage; it is often called articular (that is, of or relating to a joint) cartilage because it occurs at the ends of the articulating (opposing) bones in synovial joints. It is rather hard and translucent and is rich in collagen and proteoglycans, which help create the cellular matrix that comprises cartilage. The other primary substance in cartilage is water. Articular cartilage keeps our hard bones from rubbing against other bones and protects the soft connective tissues in our joints. For instance, when healthy, the articular cartilage of the tibia and femur of the knees slide off each other like well-oiled parts of a machine. Figure 1.1 shows the components of a healthy joint.

Articular cartilage is unusual because it does not contain any blood vessels or nerves. Because of this, cartilage grows and repairs itself more slowly than do other tissues in the body. In order for cell nourishment

Figure 1.1: The Components of a Healthy Knee Joint

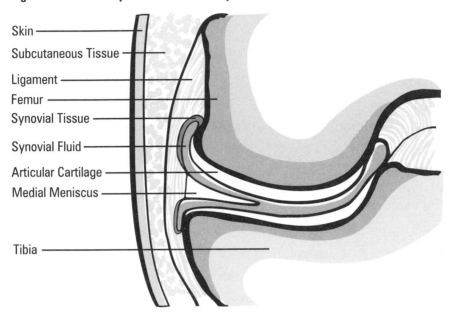

Skin
Subcutaneous Tissue
Ligament
Femur
Synovial Tissue
Synovial Fluid
Articular Cartilage
Medial Meniscus
Tibia

to support growth and repair, cartilage relies on the flexing of the joint. As the tissues in the joint move and flex, fluid that is carrying nutrients is pushed past the cartilage. The cartilage is able to absorb the nutrients through a process called diffusion (the more concentrated nutrients in the fluid pass to the cells in the cartilage where the nutrients are less concentrated). The fluid that carries the nutrients is called synovial fluid (discussed below). The nutrients, once absorbed, repair minute injuries in the cartilage and strengthen the healthy areas.

Cartilage is composed of water (65 percent to 80 percent), collagen, and proteoglycans, including chondroitin, keratan sulfate, dermatan sulfate, and hyaluronate. Collagen and the proteoglycans are produced by chondrocytes, which are specialized cells that perform specific functions throughout the body. These chondrocytes exist within the synovial tissue.

Meniscus The medial meniscus is a crescent-shaped piece of cartilage in the knee joint. It plays a critical role in knee biomechanics.

Its primary purpose is to protect the articular cartilage by acting as a shock absorber. The knees are subjected to forces of impact two to four times your body weight when you are walking and significantly greater with such high-impact activities as climbing or jogging. The meniscus contributes to joint stability and acts as a cushion between the tibia bone in the calf and the femur bone in the thigh. Loss of the meniscus through trauma, degeneration, or surgical removal has been shown to result in damage to the articular cartilage and can possibly lead to osteoarthritis.

Synovial Tissue

Synovial tissue is why the joints we're discussing are called synovial joints. Every joint is held together by ligaments, which form the joint capsule. Because the bones are not directly connected, the space between them creates a chamber. The joint capsule, or chamber, has a thin lining known as the synovial membrane (or sometimes the synovium). This membrane lines the various surfaces in the joint, including the articular cartilage, in order to reduce any friction that is caused as they rub against each other. The synovial membrane also creates a pocket, which is filled with synovial fluid.

Synovial fluid is produced by the synovial membrane and lubricates the joint capsule. The fluid creates a soft cushion between the bones, helping it function like a well-oiled machine and protecting the bones from coming in direct contact with each other. In addition, of course, it provides nutrients to the cartilage. The fluid in each joint is very minimal. In fact, the amount of synovial fluid in an adult knee joint is less than half a teaspoon. The joints that occur between the vertebrae in the spine (facet joints), which will be discussed later, are the only joints that do not contain synovial fluid.

Ligaments

Every synovial joint is held together by ligaments. The ligaments are what connect the bones of the joint to each other without the bones actually coming in contact with each other, creating what is called the joint capsule. Ligaments are tough, dense strands of connective tissue that are composed of collagen fibers. They are elastic structures, but some of the ligaments in our bodies are actually stronger than bone. In fact, there have been cases when ligaments have shortened or become inelastic and have actually broken the bones to which they were connected rather than actually tearing themselves. And although they are elastic, the role of some ligaments is, paradoxically, to prevent certain movements that would cause injury to a joint. Their strength holds the bones in place and ensures that the joints move only in the correct, injury-free way. As mentioned earlier, it's helpful to think of ligaments as large, very strong rubber bands.

> It's easiest to think of ligaments as large, very strong rubber bands.

Each joint involves multiple ligaments. For instance, the knee joint has ligaments that exist inside the joint capsule and some that exist outside of the joint capsule. The most commonly injured ligaments are the medial collateral ligament (runs along the inside of knee), the lateral collateral ligament (runs along the outside), the anterior cruciate ligament (extends from upper back to lower front of the knee, connecting the tibia and the femur), and the posterior cruciate ligament (extends from the upper front to the lower back of the knee joint, also connecting to the tibia and the femur). Other ligaments include the patellar ligament, the transverse ligament, the posterior and anterior meniscofemoral ligaments, the meniscotibial ligament, and the oblique and arcuate popliteal ligaments. Phew! And just what do all these ligaments do? They work together to keep the knee joint stable and functioning.

Tendons

Tendons are bands of connective tissue that attach muscle to bones. They are made up of tightly packed collagen fibers that are held together with specialized proteins. Unlike cartilage, tendons have ample blood vessels running through them to help their tissues grow and repair themselves on their own. There are no nerve fibers in the inner tissue of tendons, but there are nerves in the outer layers and at the point where tendons connect to muscle. Such a point involves a connective unit called the Golgi tendon organ. Tendons are covered in a protective sheath, called the synovium (just like the lining of the articular joint capsule), to protect the tendons from friction as other structures move over them.

Without tendons attaching them to bone for stability, muscles would have nothing to pull against as they contract and thus would be unable to make our various body parts move. In most instances, the connection of muscle to bone via tendons happens very near joints. Muscle tissue must cross over joints to make them functional, and it must be connected to the bones that comprise a joint.

Tendons are not only the anchors for muscles, they also work with the muscles to help us move. Tendons store energy and release it. This makes them somewhat elastic and able to act as springs. For example, the Achilles tendon in the back of the ankle stretches as you flex your foot when walking, and then it springs back as you lift your foot and returns to an unflexed (unbent) position.

Back Anatomy 101

Our backs are complex combinations of multiple moving parts. These parts involve most of the same types of tissues that you see in joints: bone, cartilage, and ligaments. They are just put together a bit differently.

The main structure of the back is the spine (see figure 1.2). Your spine extends directly from the brain and houses the spinal cord, which is the tubular bundle of nerves that is a part of the central nervous system. The spine is a column of twenty-four vertebrae, with intervertebral discs between them. At the base of the spine is a bony structure, called the sacrum, which sits in the center of the pelvis. Below the sacrum is

Figure 1.2: The Vertebrae of the Spine

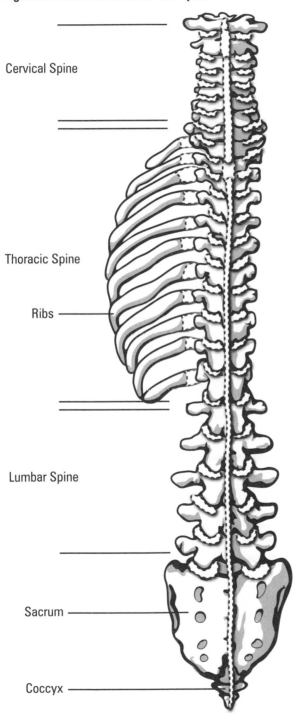

Cervical Spine

Thoracic Spine

Ribs

Lumbar Spine

Sacrum

Coccyx

the coccyx, better known as the tailbone. The spine is divided into four main sections. Going from top to bottom, they are the

- Cervical (neck area), with seven vertebrae;
- Thoracic (chest area), with twelve vertebrae;
- Lumbar (lower back area), with five vertebrae; and
- Pelvic (tailbone area), which consists of several fused sacral and coccygeal vertebrae.

Each of those sections is also referred to as a curve. Motion of the cervical, thoracic, and lumbar spines is achieved because each vertebra becomes connected with the next vertebra below it by a pair of small joints, one on each side, called facets. With overuse and aging, facets are subject to the same arthritic degeneration that affects the more visible joints, like knees, fingers, and toes. Ligaments connect portions of the spine to other bony structures.

In terms of this book, the most important aspects of the spine are (1) the intervertebral discs, and (2) the ligaments that connect the vertebrae to other structures, like the pelvis, and to each other.

As shown in figure 1.3, which is a side view of the lumbar spine and sacrum, there are a number of ligaments that help support the spinal structures and their correct positioning and movement:

- The interspinous ligaments connect adjoining vertebra.
- The ligamenta flava connect adjoining vertebra at the lamina.
- The supraspinous ligament runs from the seventh cervical vertebra to the sacrum. It connects the various vertebral joints and supports proper spinal movement.
- The anterior longitudinal ligament runs along the front of the spine (the belly side). It helps keep the vertebra and discs in proper position.
- The posterior longitudinal ligament runs along the back of the spine, through the vertebrae (through the vertebral canal), and also helps keep the vertebra and discs in proper alignment.

Figure 1.3: The Ligaments of the Spine

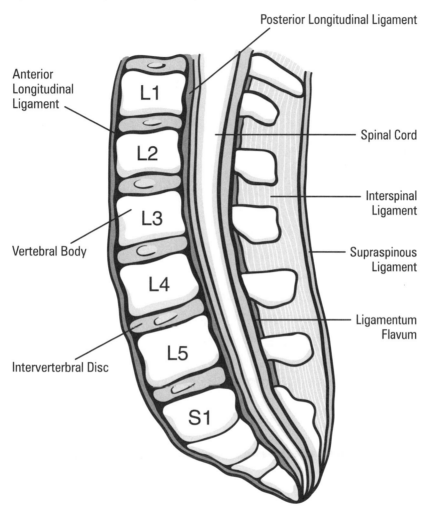

In addition to these primary ligaments, there are additional ligaments that connect the spine to other structures in the back. For example, at the top of the spine, the nuchal ligament connects the spine to the base of the skull and is an extension of the supraspinous ligament, running from the seventh cervical vertebra to the base of the skull.

For more information on the ligaments in the lower back and sacroilliac joint, refer to figure 10.5 on page 208.

Intervertebral Discs

Along with the twenty-four vertebrae, your spinal column is also composed of a series of intervertebral discs that lie between adjacent vertebrae. Each disc and the vertebrae on either side of it form a joint. Just as the meniscus absorbs forces at the knee, the intervertebral discs act as pillows to absorb or distribute forces applied to the spine (see figure 1.4). They also contribute to the stability of the spine, help maintain proper alignment of the spine, and permit movement.

You can think of intervertebral discs as tiny round gel packs. The outside of each disc is composed of a substance called fibrocartilage, which is a combination of cartilage and fibrous connective tissue. This fibrocartilage is known as the annulus fibrosus, and it is tough, flexible, and elastic. Inside of each of the discs (the nucleus pulposus) is a gel that is composed primarily of proteoglycans and water. This gel resists compression and therefore makes a good shock-absorbing center for the discs. This almost avascular (that is, lacking blood vessels) structure bears some of the greatest loads in the human body.

There are twenty-three discs in the spine, and they are named according to which vertebrae they separate (for instance, C5-6 is the disc between the fifth and sixth cervical vertebrae).

What Happens When We Are Injured?

At the young age of twenty-two, Chris had already been in pain for years. It had started when he was studying in Europe. He couldn't recall any particular event that had precipitated the pain. During his travels, he would sit on hard benches and train seats and would walk long distances while carrying a heavy backpack. At some point, his hips began to hurt. He would suddenly experience severe pain in both hips that would radiate down his legs. The pain would come on for no apparent reason, last many minutes, and resolve spontaneously. As time went on, Chris became severely limited in how far he could walk, and he could not run at all. These were serious concerns for someone his age who still desired to be active in sports and adventurous activities.

Figure 1.4: The Intervertebral Disc

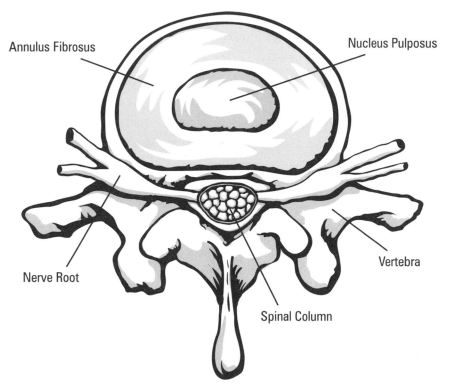

Annulus Fibrosus

Nucleus Pulposus

Nerve Root

Vertebra

Spinal Column

At first Chris consulted an orthopedist with a great reputation (he was the physician for a major college football team). When the doctor reviewed Chris's MRIs, it appeared that his hips and lower back were normal. Chris even had a total bone scan, but nothing out of the ordinary showed up. The physician referred Chris to a rheumatologist, a specialist in arthritic diseases. All of the blood tests came back negative, but because he had a scaly rash, Chris was diagnosed with psoriatic arthritis. When Chris researched the diagnosis and contested it, the doctor simply said that it made no difference because there was no additional treatment to use alongside nonsteroidal anti-inflammatory drugs (NSAIDs) anyway. Unfortunately, Chris had already been treated with NSAIDs without improvement.

Chris then went to a physical rehabilitation specialist who had a large athletic following. Since local college athletes frequently consulted this doctor, Chris believed that he would be able to locate injuries that a rheumatologist might not be used to finding. The physical rehab specialist was able to identify several tight muscle groups in Chris's back, and so they worked to relax the chronic spasms. Using manual manipulation, he was able to help Chris quite a bit. The relief, however, was short lived.

Chris's story is a classic tale of soft tissue injury. This type of injury is difficult both to diagnose and to treat, and it can be long lasting if not managed quickly and correctly. Therefore, someone who may have a soft tissue injury in or around a joint or in the back must understand how you might be injured in order to make the best decisions for your continued health. Chris, refusing to remain stuck with the pain and accept it as a part of his future, did what many are doing now—he went to the Internet for information and treatment alternatives. That is how he learned of prolotherapy and arrived at my office.

When I examined Chris, he was very tender along the bottom of his sacrum, particularly on the left side. And when I talked with Chris, he described his hips as "loose." Given his history, the results of all the tests he had undergone, the medications he had tried, and my examination, I believed Chris's pain was caused by ligament laxity. I treated his left sacrotuberous ligament first. This is the ligament that is situated in the low back part of the pelvis and connects the sacrum to the lower part of the hipbone. Chris responded very well to the treatments almost immediately, and he was gradually able to become more and more active. But the more his activities increased, the more his right hip began to bother him, so I treated his right side as well. Treating his right side finally gave him total relief. After just four months of prolotherapy treatment, he was pain free and in good health.

Chris's story is similar to that of many of the people I see on a daily basis. Their doctors can't tell them what's wrong, but they advise a treatment plan anyway. Soft tissue injuries are very common, yet most doctors know little about them, and they are not knowledgeable about all of the available ways to treat these types of injuries. Consequently, patients live in pain, don't get treatment that can heal the underlying injury, take unhelpful medications, and often undergo unnecessary surgeries that don't resolve the problem. To help you understand what may be happening in your body, let's explore the various types of soft tissue injuries that can — and often do — occur.

Sprain

You were playing with your child in the yard and you twisted your ankle. It began to swell and bruise and was painful to walk on. Your first thought was, "I broke my ankle!" So, off to the doctor you went. The doctor took X-rays, but couldn't find any broken bones. "You just have a bad sprain," she tells you. But what does that mean?

Ligaments are elastic and strong, but they can be overstretched to the point of injury. This is what doctor's mean by *sprain*. The typical signs of a sprain include inflammation, pain, swelling, and loss of function, that is, the inability to use an injured ankle, knee, wrist, or finger — the areas most likely to succumb to sprain. If your sprain does not keep you from working or doing your daily activities, you can work around it. But seriously sprain your back, neck, shoulders, knees, or hips, and you're in trouble. You'll know it's serious because the pain won't let you go about your work and daily chores. Though all of them carry the same label, sprains come in varying degrees. For example:

- A first-degree sprain involves stretching of the ligament and possibly some very minor tears. It will cause mild pain, some joint stiffness, and possibly swelling. This type of sprain typically heals well and quickly with little intervention.

- A second-degree sprain involves mild tears in the fibers of the ligament, with only minimal joint instability. This type of sprain will be more painful, will involve swelling of the joint, and can result in some instability of the joint. If you have this type of sprain, the healing process will be longer; and if you aren't careful in your treatment or how you use the joint, you could do more serious damage relatively easily.

- A third-degree sprain involves rupture of the ligament and serious joint instability. The pain is severe and is accompanied by much swelling. As the swelling increases, the pain becomes more intense, particularly if you attempt to use the joint or put weight on it. This type of sprain typically requires immediate medical treatment to ensure that the ligament heals fully and correctly.

Ligament injuries are more common than many physicians realize and can "refer" pain to distant sites. This means that although a certain ligament is injured, you may feel pain in a completely different part of the body. A specific ligament referral pattern will help your physician determine which ligaments have actually been injured. We'll discuss referred pain patterns in the next chapter.

To understand how the body attempts to protect itself from injury, recall what happens when your doctor checks your reflexes. He uses a small rubber hammer to tap against the tendon in your knee. When the tapping is done forcefully, the tendon is stretched rapidly. The body reacts quickly, sending a signal back to the spinal cord to warn the tendon against becoming overstretched and possibly torn. To prevent a tendon tear, the spinal cord sends a signal back to the muscles surrounding that joint to contract. In the case of the patellar (knee) tendon, this occurs when your leg jerks forward involuntarily. This is known as a reflex, and it can prevent the tendon from tearing.

When a ligament has been injured, it becomes weaker and looser than it was before the injury. The result is a less-stable joint. A sprained ankle, for example, will be unstable and more likely to twist again than it would have before the injury, particularly if the ligaments have not been given sufficient time to heal. Reinjury is therefore quite common. Fortunately, prolotherapy can restore function and eliminate pain by tightening overstretched and lax ligaments. The goal of prolotherapy is to restore the tissue to its normal length and strength. Doing so also restores skeletal support.

The biggest concern with sprains is the possibility that ligaments may not heal fully or correctly, and that ruptures may not heal even when sutured back together. Because of their makeup, ligaments have difficulty initiating a spontaneous healing response. That reality, combined with such other factors as delayed treatment, inappropriate treatment, and repeated injury, is likely to explain why ligament sprains often fail to heal completely. And as many of us know first-hand, when a ligament fails to heal completely, pain will occur when you move or when you hold a certain position for too long.

> When a ligament has been injured, it becomes weaker and looser than it was before the injury.

Unfortunately, when broken bones near a joint accompany soft tissue injuries, immobilizing the joint is usually necessary in order for the fracture to heal. When this happens, the patient will likely require physical rehabilitation after the bone has healed to address the soft tissue injuries and to reinvigorate the tissues in and around the joint.

In some cases of soft tissue injuries, the pain will be so intense that the patient will choose not to move the joint. As discussed, this movement is required if soft tissue injuries are to heal well and completely. Delays in physical therapy or complete lack of movement increase the likelihood that an injury will become chronic and much more difficult to resolve.

Strains and Other Muscle Injuries

Muscle injuries are generally left to heal on their own, but allowing this to happen can result in chronic spasm or contraction. Chronic muscle pain is often referred to as myofascial pain syndrome. This type of chronic pain can result from trauma or repetitive use, or it can be secondary to underlying disease. With chronic joint abnormalities, certain muscles may tighten to try to stabilize a joint junction.

Spasms occur when muscles are stretched beyond their normal range of motion and consequently tighten to protect themselves from further damage, causing muscle strain. Usually, after the threat of a muscle tear has passed, the muscle will return to its normal position; however, if a muscle tear occurs despite contraction, a chronic muscle spasm may occur. Reflex contractions of the muscle may also result from injury to the associated tendon. This may explain why many episodes of myofascial pain syndrome recur until the tendon injury is resolved. While prolotherapy does not treat muscle injuries directly, treating tendons that may be injured or weak may provide correct support for a joint and allow a spasming muscle to return to its normal state of relaxation.

People with muscle pain often have trigger points, which are sometimes called "knots." Trigger points are tender muscle cords that may transmit pain to distant sites when pressure is applied.

For many people, both the tendons and the muscles may not heal despite the body's best efforts. In such cases, normal movement must be maintained, for two key reasons: (1) Normal movement helps the body achieve a strong repair where the tendon attaches to the bone and muscle; and (2) normal movement prevents adhesions, which are inflammatory bands or scarring that joins the tendon or muscle to surrounding structures. Adhesions prevent the tendon or muscle from moving as freely as it did before the injury. In fact, scarring can cause pain upon movement or even restrict movement. Simple, nonaggressive movement during the healing process can help prevent this occurrence.

Physical rehabilitation can also help resolve any muscle atrophy, or loss of muscle tissue and strength, that results from not using the muscle for a long period of time.

Physicians commonly prescribe muscle relaxants for injuries involving tender, tight muscles. When muscle relaxants alone are not sufficient for returning the muscle to normal, massages and physical therapy are often added to the regimen. Physical therapy may consist of heat applications, stretching, and electrical stimulation or ultrasound to help loosen chronically contracted muscles. In more stubborn cases, intervention by osteopaths, chiropractors, or physical therapists specifically trained in soft tissue injuries may be required to help muscles relax. One technique these professionals are likely to employ is known as the strain–counter strain technique (which we discuss in greater detail in chapter 6). This involves stretching the muscle to its proper length and holding it for a few seconds to help reeducate the muscle in finding its proper position. Such stretching techniques may also break adhesions within the muscle bed itself.

When muscle spasms become chronic and unrelieved by the usual methods, the patient generally describes a constant feeling of achiness, tightness, and pain with movement. Pain medicines are not very effective in relieving these symptoms. When a muscle spasm becomes chronic, relief can be challenging, if achievable. In later chapters, we discuss some of the various types of treatments that are available for people with chronic muscle spasms, including the use of botulinum toxin.

Tendon Injuries and Conditions

Among the various types of injuries and conditions associated with tendons are tears, tendinitis, and tendinosis. When the tendon is injured, using its associated muscle will be excruciating. Active therapy for any associated muscle issues has to be delayed until the tendon is healed. Only gentle stretching techniques can be used initially.

If a tendon is stretched beyond its range, the tendon can tear in any one of three places: where it joins to the bone, where it joins to the muscle, or at the midsection of the tendon itself. Because the tendon is stronger than the bone or muscle to which it is attached, making tears to the midsection is the least common of these injuries. When the bone is broken from the tendon, it is referred to as an avulsion fracture, a condition that often requires surgery.

Tendinitis is the irritation and inflammation of a tendon, typically as a result of overuse. As we become older or if we are inactive, it becomes easier to injure our tendons and other soft tissues because they are not well conditioned for sudden bouts of activity. Tendinitis is most common in the shoulders, elbows, wrists, and heels. Common symptoms of tendinitis include pain (usually very close to but just outside of the related joint), tenderness, and mild swelling. Many people who experience these symptoms self-treat with over-the-counter anti-inflammatory medicines. Unfortunately, that could be the worse thing for the healing process, as I'll explain in detail in later chapters.

The symptoms of tendinosis mirror those of tendinitis and can include pain on use, tenderness, and swelling and inflammation. In fact, tendinosis is often thought of as chronic tendinitis, but recent research has found that this is not an accurate assumption. Tendinosis is damage to a tendon at a cellular level, which causes the fraying or degeneration of the fibers of the tendon. Although most medical practitioners are taught that tendon pain is most likely attributable to tendinitis (at least upon a patient's first visit), tendinosis is actually the more likely and more accurate diagnosis in many cases (Khan et al., 2002). Furthermore, the usual treatment prescribed for tendinitis will not help with tendinosis.

Tenosynovitis is the inflammation of the sheath that surrounds a tendon. The lining of the sheath, as you might recall, is the synovium; thus, the name of the condition. This condition can result from injury, strain, or overuse, but it can also result from infection. The symptoms are pain, stiffness, inflammation, and swelling of a joint. Fever and redness may indicate an infection; in such an instance, you should see your doctor immediately. Tenosynovitis is most commonly seen in the wrists, hands, and feet.

If a tendon injury or condition does not heal correctly or if it is not treated properly, the tissue surrounding the tendon can become permanently scarred and thus lock the tendon in place, preventing movement. This is a problem particularly in smaller joints, such as the finger joints.

I want to point out that tendinitis, tendinosis, and tenosynovitis can also be caused by repetitive use or overuse—factors that are discussed in detail in the next section.

Repetitive Stress or Strain Injuries, Overuse Syndromes, and Cumulative Trauma Disorders

Many different types of syndromes are commonly associated with repetitive use of a limb or a joint, and the majority of them affect the soft tissues surrounding a joint. While the terms repetitive stress injuries, overuse syndromes, and cumulative trauma disorders are used as catchalls for these syndromes or conditions, each is uniquely different depending on the part of the body involved, the symptoms, and other factors. What they do have in common, however, is that they can result from any of the following situations:

- Thousands of repetitive movements daily that involve little force, such as typing
- Dozens of daily movements involving greater force, such as lifting heavy loads or other types of intense manual labor
- Improper posture that results in misuse or mispositioning of the trunk of the body and limbs

That said, not all evidence fully supports the idea that carpal tunnel syndrome, tennis elbow, golfer's elbow, and other similar conditions are caused by repetitive use. Other factors may be involved, such as physical abnormalities or improper healing from a previous injury. When an injury has occurred to the soft tissue surrounding a joint, the last thing you should do is stop moving. Lack of movement can quickly cause greater damage due to reduced blood flow and other elements critical to tissue repair and regeneration.

> When an injury has occurred to the soft tissue surrounding a joint, the last thing you should do is stop moving.

The following paragraphs briefly describe some of the most common conditions that fall within this category of injury. Symptoms common to most of these conditions include pain, swelling, inflammation, tenderness, stiffness, and weakness or lack of endurance:

- *Carpal tunnel syndrome*: This condition occurs when the median nerve that runs from the forearm into the hand becomes compressed by the carpal tunnel—a rigid passage of ligament and bones at the base of the hand. The tunnel may become constricted by pressure from irritated tendons or swelling from other soft tissues. Because the nerve is being affected, a common symptom is numbness or tingling in the palm of the hand near the wrist or thumb. According to the National Institutes of Health, surgery for carpal tunnel syndrome, in which the carpal ligament is severed and the tunnel is opened, is one of the most common surgical procedures currently performed in the United States.

- *Tennis elbow*: Also called lateral epicondylitis, this condition involves the inflammation and possible degeneration of the tendon in the forearm that connects to the lateral epicondyle, that is, the bulge at the end of the humerus (upper arm bone) that you can feel on the outside of your elbow. The pain associated with this condition often radiates from the outside of the elbow, down the forearm, to the back of the hand, particularly when a person is grasping or twisting an object.

- *Golfer's elbow*: This condition is very similar to tennis elbow except that it affects the inside of the elbow. It is also called medial epicondylitis because that is the point of connection between the humerus and the tendon that extends into the forearm.

- *Trigger finger*: This condition is a form of tenosynovitis. The sheath around the tendon in the affected finger becomes irritated, and eventually the sheath narrows to the point that it prohibits movement and causes the finger to become locked in a bent position.

- *Bursitis*: This condition is caused by the inflammation of the bursas in a joint. A bursa is a small, fluid-filled sac between a tendon and a bone that provides cushioning and reduces friction. When a joint is overused, the bursa can become irritated and inflamed. This condition is most common in the shoulders and elbows.

Repetitive strain injury (RSI) is also sometimes used to describe a condition that seems to result from repetitive use of a limb, particularly the arms. This condition does not have a singular, specific soft tissue problem related to it that can be detected. Instead, the pain is typically more diffuse, possibly covering the entire arm, and there may be muscle spasms as well. Other symptoms include pain that worsens with activity, inflammation, stiffness, weakness or lack of endurance, and nerve pain.

Dislocation

Every joint is held firmly in position by the articular capsule that is primarily made up of ligaments. When a limb is under severe pressure during trauma, the bones associated with a joint can pop out of the joint capsule and become misaligned. The ligaments that form the capsule are thus traumatized and may be seriously injured. The first step in treating a dislocation is to "reduce" the joint back into its normal position. This is typically done manually, pulling the limb away from the joint and then angling the misaligned bone back into its correct position. This process can be very painful, but once a dislocation has been corrected, healing of the surrounding soft tissues can begin.

Young, healthy individuals have more-flexible ligaments than older people, which means their ligaments may be able to stretch without tearing or being seriously injured. During a dislocation, therefore, older individuals will probably tear a ligament or two. This more severe injury to the ligaments may set the joint up for chronic dislocation, that is, it easily becomes dislocated again and again. Maintaining ligament and tendon flexibility is very important both in limiting further injury or preventing it altogether.

Subluxation

A subluxation is a partial dislocation of a joint. With subluxations, the trauma to the surrounding ligaments may be less severe than with full dislocations. Nevertheless, most of the same issues regarding treatment, such as the need for immediate reduction of the joint into proper position, still exist.

In chiropractic medicine and other manual medicines, subluxation refers to the improper alignment or juxtaposition of vertebrae with the surrounding vertebrae. Weak ligaments allow the vertebrae to move out of position. This results in pain both around the spine and in the referred patterns throughout the body (see the information on referred pain patterns in the next chapter). Improving your posture or chiropractic adjustment may provide relief. If the ligaments remain weak, though, prolotherapy can help make the relief permanent.

Cartilage Tears

Cartilage tears can occur in almost any joint in the body as a result of trauma or overuse of a joint. As part of the aging process, cartilage begins to break down; therefore, cartilage tears can occur more easily in older men and women. Cartilage tears are probably most common in the meniscus of the knee.

The common symptoms of cartilage tears are pain in the joint, immediate swelling, limited range of motion in the joint, audible popping or clicking sounds, or the joint locking into certain positions. We'll discuss some treatments in chapters 7 and 8 that may help repair cartilage tears. Just like herniated discs, you can have cartilage tears without pain. Sometimes they require surgery, especially if a loose piece of cartilage interferes with movement of the joint.

Synovitis

Synovitis is the term used for inflammation of the synovium, particularly the synovial membrane. This inflammation may be the result of inflammatory or even noninflammatory joint diseases. Synovitis may result in swelling in and around the joint that is visible to the naked eye. This disease will alter the function of the synovium, which will affect the health of the cartilage because the synovial fluid will not be replenished with nutrients as it should be. The volume, viscosity, and white blood cell count in the synovial fluid will be affected.

Spinal Injuries and Conditions

Pain in the lower back is one of the most common forms of chronic pain. It can be caused by a number of factors, from injuries and poor conditioning of muscles and ligaments to the effects of aging or arthritis. Less-common causes of low back pain include tumors, specific inflammatory conditions, and specific diseases of bone, muscle, or nervous tissue. It comes as a surprise to many patients with chronic back pain that in more than half of the reported cases, the anatomical structure causing the pain cannot be determined with precision. In this situation—sometimes diagnosed as nonspecific back pain—it is nonetheless important to exclude potentially serious conditions. Many cases of nonspecific low back pain may result from chronic injury to ligaments and muscles.

The muscles of the lower back provide power and strength for such ordinary activities as standing, walking, and lifting. As I've already mentioned, a strain of any muscle can occur when that muscle is poorly conditioned or overworked. The ligaments and muscles of the lower back act in concert to interconnect the vertebral bones and thus provide support or stability. A sprain of the lower back can occur when a sudden, forceful movement injures a ligament that has become stiff or weak through overuse. Sometimes an individual initially even overlooks the injury. With time, however, a combination of other factors may increase and maintain the likelihood of a back injury and therefore the duration of the pain. Among those factors are continued improper use of the low back muscles, balance or gait problems, associated neurological problems that cause rigidity or weakness, obesity, or smoking.

Pain originating in the facets and sacroiliac joints may be the most underdiagnosed roots of low back pain. Pain from the SI joint is frequently localized to the buttock, but it may spread into the legs.

Without additional studies, it is often misdiagnosed as nerve root pain. This diagnosis is based primarily on a physical examination during which certain exam maneuvers are performed. The patient's responses to those maneuvers alert the pain specialist to the possibility of pain from the SI joints. That diagnosis is then confirmed by injecting local anesthetics into the joint itself using image-guided procedures. Typically, however, the X-ray or MRI appearance of the joints has little correlation to the degree of pain and does not contribute to the diagnosis. In addition, pain from a degenerated low back disc can resemble the pain that originates in the SI joint but, in contrast to popular belief, the degenerated disc is far less commonly the source of such pain.

Skeletal irregularities produce strain on the vertebrae and supporting muscles, tendons, ligaments, and tissues supported by the spinal column. These irregularities include scoliosis, a curving of the spine to the side; kyphosis, in which the normal curve of the upper back is severely rounded; lordosis, an abnormally accentuated arch in the lower back; back extension, a bending backward of the spine; and back flexion, in which the spine bends forward.

Disc Injuries and Conditions

A number of disc conditions can cause back pain or affect mobility. Among these conditions are bulging discs, herniated discs, and degenerative disorders. As described earlier, our discs are like little gel packs, with a thick outer container called the annulus fibrosus and a soft inner core called the nucleus pulposus (see figure 1.4). When a disc is bulging, the annulus fibrosus has become weak and is bulging outward. If that weakened point ruptures, releasing the nucleus pulposus, the disc is said to be herniated, or ruptured (see figure 1.5).

Two main types of pain can result from the degeneration of a disc: One type of pain comes from inside the disc itself (called discogenic pain); the other type comes from disc herniation, which can compress a nearby spinal nerve. Disc damage, or degeneration, can occur as an ongoing process caused by repetitive trauma or aging, in which water

Figure 1.5: Herniated and Bulging Discs

Prolapsed Disc

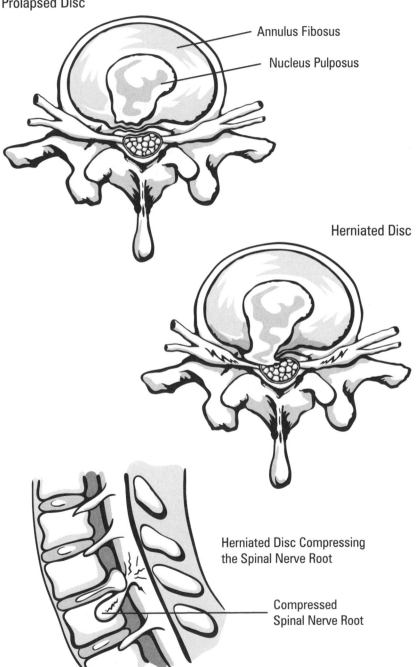

Annulus Fibosus

Nucleus Pulposus

Herniated Disc

Herniated Disc Compressing
the Spinal Nerve Root

Compressed
Spinal Nerve Root

content decreases and abnormal fibrous tissue increases. Ultimately, the disc's load-bearing capacity is overwhelmed, leading to tears, more abnormal fibrosis, and the growth of highly vascular reparative tissue called granulation tissue into the substance of the disc itself.

In the past, there was a widespread belief that because discs were avascular, they also lacked nerves and therefore could not be the source of pain. More recently, however, careful dissections and microscopic examinations of normal and abnormal discs have led to the discovery of pain-specific nerve terminals, called C nerve fibers, within the substance of normal intervertebral discs themselves. Furthermore, degenerated discs were found to exhibit an abnormal proliferation of these pain-generating nerve terminals, potentially making them more prone to cause pain than normal discs. During middle age, the nucleus of each disc starts losing water and the annulus fibrosus starts bearing the burden of spine motion and trauma, no longer cushioned by the nucleus pulposus. The end results are fissures, or cracks, in the annulus. These may be the source of back pain because the C fibers exist only in the annulus. Pain that originates from degenerated discs can range from mild to unbearable, yet autopsy and clinical studies have demonstrated that, surprisingly, even though degenerated discs are common in middle age and more so in old age, they are not always accompanied by pain.

The other significant form of pain involving a disc results from compression of a nerve living in the vicinity of a degenerated disc. Sometimes tears in the annulus of the disc allow the softer center to come out, which leads to compression of a nearby spinal nerve root. The common terms for this condition are a disc bulge, or bulging disc, and a herniated disc. When the herniated disc presses a nerve, it may cause pain in the leg, which is frequently referred to as sciatica. Often, an associated inflammation appears in the area of compression that can be alleviated with treatment (see figure 1.4).

As discussed later, some people have disc problems, yet they have no symptoms. Other people have disc problems and a variety of symptoms that may include nerve pain and limited motion. Some disc problems may require surgery to resolve, but in some cases, surgery will not be helpful. In many cases, disc problems may occur because the vertebrae of the spine are out of proper alignment because of the laxity of the surrounding ligaments. In these cases, prolotherapy can be especially helpful.

How We Heal

When we injure ourselves, our body immediately responds by starting the healing cascade. This is the process our bodies go through to identify injured cells, remove those that are damaged, and generate new cells to replace those that were damaged. It is a truly amazing process and an area of science where new discoveries are made all the time.

The healing of an injury can be separated into three distinct phases:

1. *The inflammatory phase*: This is the phase that causes pain. There are actually two stages to the inflammatory phase: The early stage typically lasts about three days. The late phase typically lasts about ten days. In the early inflammatory process, chemicals are released to attract granulocytes and macrophages, which are types of white blood cells. These will simultaneously clear out the dead and injured tissue in order to prepare the area for repair and secrete growth factors, which will attract and activate fibroblasts. These activated fibroblasts will lay down new collagen, which is the structural material that gives strength to the tendons and ligaments. In the cascade of events that leads to the healing of a torn ligament or tendon, five substances are initially released to the injured site in a cascade effect to further the healing process:

   • Cytokines support the formation of chemokines and growth factors.

- Chemokines act to draw other important cells to the area.
- Arachidonic acid (an Omega-6 fatty acid) helps generate prostaglandins and leukotrienes.
- Growth factors promote cell proliferation.
- Catabolic enzymes break down the extracellular matrix so that the injured cells can be released.

2. *Granulation tissue formation*: During this phase injured or dead tissue, which was removed, is replaced with healthy living cells. Granulation tissue is made up of fibroblasts, which were drawn to the wound by chemicals secreted during the inflammatory phase.

3. *Matrix formation and remodeling*: During this phase the granulation tissue matures into the normal tissue. The fibroblasts form collagen, which is the primary component of ligament and tendon fibers. The tensile strength of the tendon and ligaments slowly returns as the healing is completed. As the tissue matures the inflammatory cells decrease in number.

All healing processes in the body begin with inflammation, whether it is caused by trauma or a bacterial infection. Whenever you injure yourself the body automatically begins an inflammatory response. The swelling you see when you twist your ankle, for example, is part of an inflammatory response. You would not be able to heal the ligament sprain without the inflammation. Yet the average person has been led to believe that inflammation is bad. Just think of all of the anti-inflammatory medications you probably have in your medicine cabinet.

When inflammation occurs when you twist your ankle, it is beneficial and it has a beginning and an end. It is not a bad thing. Chronic inflammation, however, is a totally different story. This type of inflammation can be very detrimental, and depending on the cause, typically requires treatment. An acute inflammatory response is your friend. A chronic inflammatory response is your enemy.

Arthritic Changes

Arthritis is a leading cause of productivity loss. The most common form associated with degenerated joints is osteoarthritis, which affects more than half of adults over sixty-five and is more likely to affect women than men. Arthritis pain occurs because of the breakdown of cartilage, which results from wear and tear, injury, obesity, and broken bones. If you have a parent or relative who suffers from arthritis, you are also more likely to develop it. Arthritis is associated with morning stiffness or stiffness after exercise, pain accompanying movement, cracking, swelling, and redness of joints, and loss of flexibility. Arthritis of the facets, also called degenerative joint disease of the spine, facet arthropathy, or spondylosis, can be debilitating. Facet arthritis can be the cause of low back pain in up to 40 percent of patients over fifty years of age. Cervical facets may contribute to pain in up to 30 percent of cases who complain of chronic headaches.

There is no cure for arthritis. Thus, the mainstream therapeutic goal of treatment for osteoarthritis is to minimize the effects of the disease and its consequences over time and to teach patients how to self-manage it.

Typical changes associated with arthritis are loosening of the joints, hypermobility, and ligament incompetence. These conditions allow the joint to move in ways that it should not, extending too far in any one direction. This increases the risk of further injury. To help the joints remain stable, the muscles overcompensate (when they are able) and this causes muscle pain. Although these changes cannot be undone, further damage can be minimized and the pain associated with arthritis can be lessened. A trip to the doctor's office usually results in a prescription for a nonsteroidal anti-inflammatory medication (NSAID). But NSAIDs often fail to relieve pain, and they come with a host of side effects that can be more damaging and painful than the arthritis itself.

To alleviate arthritis pain, I recommend rest, massage, exercise (particularly nonweight-bearing exercises), and sometimes prolotherapy.

In most cases, your physician will tell you there is no complete healing from arthritis; you have to live with the pain. Prolotherapy, however, can play a role in repairing arthritic joints in some patients. It has proven to be useful in relieving pain where there is excessive joint movement.

Rheumatoid arthritis is a chronic and progressively degenerative and inflammatory condition in which the immune system attacks its own joints (thus, it is considered an autoimmune disorder). Rheumatoid arthritis affects joint tissue as well as tissues throughout the body involving the skin, blood vessels, heart, lungs, and muscles. This is not a condition that prolotherapy can treat because of the chronic inflammation that already exists.

Defining your pain, its location, and its cause are key elements in the healing process. To do this, you need to understand how your joints and spine function and how injuries affect these critical parts of your body. With this knowledge, you can begin to take action to stop your pain or to heal your injury.

Chapter 2

Understanding Your Pain

Mike is a middle-aged physical education teacher. During the fall of 2004, he participated in his town's popular annual YMCA Dragon Boat Races, an all-day athletic extravaganza that included rowing, volleyball, tug-of-war, and dodgeball. Many local businesses, churches, and schools organized their own teams. While playing in an elimination round of dodgeball, Mike felt a *pop* in the inside of his right elbow. He managed to finish the game, but with an intense burning and stabbing pain in his arm. After six weeks of self-treating his injury with rest, massage, and anti-inflammatory medication, he finally decided to see an orthopedic surgeon.

Pain is something many of us deal with on a daily basis. Some people just accept it as a fact of life. We think it will eventually get better or we believe that we can live with it. But pain causes an enormous amount of stress on the body, and stress in itself is detrimental to your health. Even one small injury can affect your sleep, your eating habits, your work, and your overall contentment with life.

Now that you've read chapter 1, you have a much better understanding of the type of injury you're experiencing and how the parts of your body work together. This is important information to grasp. But you are also probably in pain, and therefore you need to understand your pain, too, and what you can do about it. To help you with this critical next step, I'm going to describe different types of pain that people experience and the most common sources of each type. Then I'm going to walk you through an initial visit with a doctor.

Types and Levels of Pain

Pain is considered to be a multidimensional symptom. What this means is that many diverse factors can increase or decrease pain, beyond the extent of the actual injury. For chronic pain patients, obtaining relief from their symptoms is sometimes difficult because there are different contributors, and each needs to be treated specifically. Patients are often sent back and forth between specialists of all kinds in search of a solution.

To help you better understand your pain, I'll describe two types of pain—somatic and neuropathic pain—and two levels of pain—acute pain and chronic pain—and some of the dimensions that contribute to each.

Somatic and Neuropathic Pain

There are several types of pain, but somatic and neuropathic are the types most frequently associated with back or joint injuries. Somatic pain, in particular, is the type of pain you are most likely experiencing.

Somatic pain, particularly deep somatic pain, occurs when tissues—ligaments, tendons, muscle, bones, and fascia—are damaged in some way. The nociceptors—sensory receptors in the form of nerve endings—in the area actually react to the mechanical, thermal, or chemical changes that are occurring. They initiate the signal to the brain, which registers the changes and then initiates a pain response.

There are not many pain receptors in the deeper tissues of the body, so somatic pain tends to be a diffuse, dull, aching pain rather than sharp or very localized. Somatic pain is often associated with the inflammatory healing response, which is why NSAIDs are used to treat it.

Neuropathic pain may occur when there is no sign of the original injury, yet the nerves continue to send messages to the brain about tissue damage. In this condition, damaged nerves misfire and send incorrect signals to other pain centers, changing nerve function at the site of injury or nearby areas. The original injury sets up a pathway in the nervous system and sends a pain signal even though there is no tissue damage. Your brain is triggered to feel pain, though the pain point or cause may be impossible to locate.

Neuropathic pain may be caused by amputation, chemotherapy, diabetes, HIV infection, multiple sclerosis, shingles, or surgery, particularly spinal surgery. The pain manifests as either burning or tingling or numbness. Patients who have had limbs amputated can still experience pain from the nerves that originally carried impulses from the limb. This type of pain does not respond well to treatment and people are often told to take medications indefinitely. Over time, neuropathic pain can worsen and require even greater doses of pain killing medication. Unfortunately, prolotherapy does not alleviate neuropathic pain.

Acute Pain

Getting injured is part of life; most of us experience small-scale injuries on a regular basis. You may touch a hot pan, stub your toe, smash your finger with a hammer, or step on a nail. Though painful, these injuries don't last very long or cause permanent damage. Doctors call the pain associated with these injuries acute pain, and it is generally a result of the inflammatory process that occurs when we are injured, meaning that it is generally somatic pain. Soft tissue injuries—such as an abnormal forceful stretch or tear of a ligament or a muscle by trauma, heavy lifting, or a fall—also cause acute pain, at least initially. Acute pain usually lasts anywhere from a few days to six months, until the injured tissue has healed. Once the tissue is completely healed, the pain should be gone. The danger with soft tissue injuries is that they might never fully heal and the pain might never completely disappear.

Besides the time frame, another distinct characteristic of acute pain is that you can always locate the root of the pain. If you touch a hot pan, the source, or location, of the pain is your burned fingertips. If you twist your ankle and sprain it, you'll feel the pain in your ankle. It is easy to diagnose acute pain and to identify the area that is causing the pain.

Many of the injuries associated with acute pain will heal on their own and do not require surgery or any special medical services. Yet acute pain is one of the main reasons why people seek emergency or urgent care. Emergency room doctors often see people in acute pain that results from soft tissue damage. But for the most part, their job is to ensure that there are no broken bones or nerve injuries, address the comfort of the patient as the body naturally heals, and control the pain associated with the injury.

Unfortunately, patients who seek help in the emergency room do not always receive adequate amounts of medication to relieve their pain. Several studies have reported that patients often still have high levels of pain when they are discharged (Ducharme and Barber, 1995; Johnston et al., 1998; Todd et al., 2002, 2007). If treated correctly, patients should leave the facility with their pain under control and a working knowledge of how to continue to aid the natural healing process, whether that be elevation, ice packs, or heat compressions. Deficiencies in the treatment of acute pain have recently led to the development of practical guidelines to improve the quality of care in emergency rooms.

When acute pain isn't treated quickly and appropriately, there are two possible results: (1) The pain becomes established and is therefore more difficult to treat or suppress. In other words, the longer pain remains in an injured area, the deeper it becomes and the harder it is to relieve. (2) The pain progresses from acute pain to chronic pain. Acute pain can become chronic for a variety of reasons, among them progression of a disease (such as arthritis), a chronic infection, repetitive trauma, or the persistence of the abnormalities caused by the disease or injury after the initial condition has resolved.

Insufficient care in emergency rooms is responsible for causing many cases of acute pain, which should have resolved fairly quickly, to develop into chronic pain. The only way to prevent acute pain from becoming chronic is to make sure that the injury that caused the pain heals fully and correctly. When acute pain isn't treated appropriately and lingers, the limitations on normal and pleasurable activities, together with anxiety that results from the pain itself, can cause depression, making the situation worse and delaying the natural healing process.

> To prevent acute pain from becoming chronic, make sure that the injury that caused the pain heals fully and correctly.

Chronic Pain

Pain that lasts longer than three to six months or beyond the point when tissue has healed is called chronic pain. The area seems to have healed or at least looks so to the naked eye or even under basic examination, but for some reason the pain remains. Maybe the initial injury wasn't treated appropriately and healed poorly as a result; maybe the injury was more severe than you or your doctor originally thought; maybe you reinjured the soft tissues. Chronic pain can be either somatic (particularly from a condition that causes chronic inflammation) or neuropathic.

Obviously, the biggest concern with chronic pain is lack of comfort. But the related effects are also extremely important to consider. One major concern is that chronic pain can, and often does, cause long-term changes in your body. For example, if you have long-term pain in your right knee, you will probably walk favoring that leg. This causes the muscles in the left leg to strengthen and the muscles in the right leg will weaken. Though physical therapy can attempt to restore a balance, many chronic pain injuries cause changes in the body that can never be fully restored. (As mentioned in the story of Andres in chapter 1, prolotherapy is a great way to help strengthen and restore balance to the body.)

It is impossible to identify when chronic pain begins (because it never actually begins as chronic pain), therefore much less is known about it than about acute pain. (In chapter 10, you'll read about Ollie who didn't realize her chronic pain originated from her car accident fifty years earlier.) Sometimes, chronic pain is caused by an identifiable pain generator, such as an injury, a structural problem in a joint or the back, or a disease. For instance, certain structural conditions, such as degenerative disc disease or spinal stenosis, can cause ongoing pain until treatment has been provided. Whether the pain began in child-hood or its onset occurred when the person was older, chronic pain will remain, and possibly increase, until it is treated effectively. Still other times, chronic pain can be rooted in a soft tissue injury that went untreated or was treated poorly.

A large percentage of visits to primary care physicians involve chronic pain, more specifically, chronic pain that resulted from mus-culoskeletal injuries. These types of injuries involve muscles and the parts of the skeleton they surround and support. Given the intricacy of the human body and the vast number of muscles and bones that affect each other, it is not surprising that a bone injury can morph into a musculoskeletal injury if proper attention is not given to it.

One of the components that is unrelated to the pain generator, yet plays a large role in the experience of pain, is called pain centralization. This is a name given to a process whereby there is an abnormal activation of certain nerve cells in the brain and spinal cord (the central nervous system) that maintain and even augment the sensation of pain. This is somewhat related to neuropathic pain, but neuropathic pain tends to be associated with the peripheral nervous system (damage to the nerves at the site of trauma). Studies have not been conclusive about how the two relate to or differ from each other (Devor, 2006).

One example of a condition associated with pain centralization is phantom limb syndrome; in this situation, the patient experiences pain although a limb has been amputated. Brain circuitries abnormally maintain or even increase the level of perceived pain in an arm or a leg that is no longer there. Research has demonstrated that various degrees of pain centralization may affect not only those patients who underwent a limb amputation but also patients afflicted by many forms of chronic pain, such as low back pain, arthritis, neuropathy, or chronic headaches. To achieve effectiveness in the treatment of pain, each component contributing to the pain experience — for instance, pain centralization — must be addressed differently from the treatment delivered to the primary pain generator.

Even with chronic pain, there is frequently a cause. No pain is sourceless. But unlike getting bitten by a dog on your right thumb, where or how your chronic pain originated is hard to identify. What you do know when you are in chronic pain, however, is that a part of your body isn't functioning correctly. And with this realization comes the hope that you may actually be able to identify and resolve the underlying physical problem. Nevertheless, it is difficult to feel hopeful when you're in chronic pain. Depression and anxiety set in from the loss of physical ability, independence, and the simple pleasures in life. Being in low spirits adds to your stress level and hinders your body's healing or its response to medical treatment.

Identifying the Source of the Pain — The Pain Generator

When you see a doctor about your pain, he or she will want to know about the cause and source of your pain. By definition, the cause of pain is that thing that is making the pain occur — the pain generator, as described previously. This could be something as simple as a bee sting or as complex as degenerative disc disease. Though the cause of pain may be difficult to identify when it is chronic, it is still vital to try so that complete healing can be achieved. The source of pain is the area where the pain originates. For example, you may be experiencing pain in your heel, but you know that you injured your knee recently. The knee injury may be causing the heel pain; consequently, treating the heel, though important, will not entirely alleviate the pain or ensure that the heel pain will not return. In order to do that, the physician must go to the source of the pain—the knee injury.

A thorough physical and neurologic examination is considered the gold standard for identifying the anatomical structure primarily responsible for your pain. It is important that the physician identifies correctly the neuropathic or inflammatory mechanisms underlying a patient's pain because the medications and strategies used to treat each of these are different. Once a potential pain generator is suspected, confirmation of the precise structure involved can be achieved by several methods. One method that pain specialists commonly use is numbing the pain generator (or the nerves that carry pain signals from the structure) using a local anesthetic like lidocaine. Identifying and treating the pain generator are crucial to decreasing pain. These steps are also relevant to interrupting the self-perpetuating cycle contributing to pain centralization and chronicity. For this purpose, the pain physician uses high-precision injection techniques guided by such imaging methods as fluoroscopy or computerized tomography (CT).

Once a particular pain generator is identified—a painful disc or a joint in the patient's lower back, for example—it can be treated in a more-specific manner. Specialized testing may be needed, including an MRI or a nerve and muscle study (electromyography), to help the doctor determine the primary cause or mechanism of the pain. (Tests are discussed in chapter 4.) In many cases, there is no relationship between the intensity of the pain and the extent of the injury or the degree of abnormalities present in an MRI or CT scan study. Conversely, many individuals with profound abnormalities detected by these imaging techniques have little pain or no symptoms at all.

Therefore, these studies should never be interpreted in isolation (that is, without clinical correlation).

As an example, let's look at back pain that a doctor suspects to be related to a disc injury or condition. A definite diagnosis can be difficult. This is because there are no specific signs in the physical exam or imaging changes in the MRI or CT scan that can lead to an accurate diagnosis. In addition, the specific painful disc may be hard to identify because the pain originating from a single disc can extend to several levels of the spine. Diagnosis in these cases uses a method called provocative discography, which involves stressing the disc by injecting dye into it using imaging guidance at a very specific and controlled pressure. The stressing test should reproduce the pain. As pressure is applied by the doctor, only painful discs reproduce the patient's usual pain. The test has three possible outcomes: It could cause no pain; it could produce pain that is dissimilar to the patient's usual pain; or it could reproduce the usual pain. This technique guides the pain physician or surgeon in accurately targeting the painful disc for treatment.

Referred Pain Patterns

In your efforts to better understand your pain and what it may mean, it is important for you to also understand referred pain patterns. Many soft tissue injuries have referred pain patterns — that is, the pain is actually referred to (or hurts at) a site on the body other than where the injury originates. Recall the illustration earlier of a heel pain whose source was actually an injured knee. Knowing about these patterns can help identify the source of your pain. This is not a straightforward process, however, because what begins as an acute injury in one area is often misdiagnosed and becomes a chronic injury years later.

This problem of referred pain patterns stems from the fact that many soft tissue injuries involve several different types of tissue. Various ligaments may be affected by one injured ligament, for instance. And severe muscle spasms often result from soft tissue injuries, further complicating the picture.

In our daily efforts to maintain normal posture and movement, mild stress is placed on ligaments, and there is usually little muscle contraction. But when an injury occurs, the resulting ligament laxity causes joint instability. This puts more of the burden on your muscles to maintain normal posture and movement. After a period of time, muscle spasms develop. A spasming muscle is usually a sign of underlying injury, not the primary cause of the pain. Holding your arm out in front of you is easy for a short while; holding it there for an hour will result in severe pain and muscle spasm. Thus, putting undue stress on muscles comes with a price — pain and spasm.

> Most physicians are not as knowledgeable about the referred pain patterns caused by soft tissue injuries.

Most physicians are extremely aware of referred nerve pain patterns called dermatomal pain. What most physicians are not as knowledgeable about, however, are the referred pain patterns caused by soft tissue injuries, or scleratomal pain patterns. Each pattern is specific to different ligament strains — hence, the difficulty of diagnosing and treating soft tissue injuries.

The areas of the body that are sources of referred pain are shoulders, neck, thorax, lower back, sacrum, buttocks, and hip joints — core structures close to the spine and center of the nervous system. The structures further from the body's core do not typically radiate pain to other areas. This has much to do with how various parts of the body are linked through the nervous and other systems.

Ben E. Benjamin, author of the 1984 bestseller *Listen to Your Pain*, outlined several givens in any discussion of referred pain patterns in an article published in 2006. Among them are the following three principles, which can help any doctor identify the area of original injury:

1. Pain refers away from the core of the body, out toward the extremities.

2. Referred pain does not cross the midline of the body (an injury on the left side does not refer pain to the right side).

3. The distance of the referred pain from the point of injury reflects the severity of the injury.

LIGAMENT REFERRED PAIN PATTERNS

- A ligament injury in the lumbar spine can result in radiating pain down the leg to the knee.
- A ligament injury to the shoulder may refer pain to the upper arm or, if more severe, down to the wrist.
- Ligament laxity at the top of the cervical spine, where it connects to the occipital bone, can refer pain to the forehead, eyes, temple, and above the ear.
- A sprained or weakened ligament in the cervical spine (neck) can refer pain to the shoulder and down the arm, all the way to the fingers.
- A ligament problem in the hip, particularly where the femur sits in the hip joint, can refer pain to the front and outside areas of the lower leg.
- Ligament laxity in the sacroiliac (SI) joint can refer pain to the outside, or lateral, lower leg.

Other Factors Contributing to Pain

Pain, as mentioned at the beginning of this chapter, is considered to be a multidimensional symptom. We have defined some of those dimensions already, including the pain generator and the possible centralization of pain. Three other influential factors to consider are the link between pain and mental health, how pain is tied to physical conditioning or deconditioning, and the link between pain and related illnesses or conditions.

Pain and Mental Health An important example of the multidimensional nature of pain is the presence of associated mood abnormalities, such as depression. Mood is regulated in the brain by the same molecules (mainly norepinephrine and serotonin) that are implicated in pain tolerance. The levels of these substances frequently diminish in chronic pain, which can lead not only to a vicious cycle of decreased pain tolerance but also to chronic depression, a condition characterized by persistent feelings of low mood and loss of interest or pleasure in usual activities. Interestingly, the reverse is also true: Patients afflicted by depression are more susceptible to developing chronic pain. Thus, if the treating physician determines that depression is contributing to the patient's experience of pain, it is critical that additional treatments (pharmacologic and psychological) be prescribed to address the painful condition. Such treatment does not imply that the patients' pain "comes only from their head" in the psychiatric sense. For some people, pain and mood can improve substantially after they are prescribed an antidepressant medication that increases the levels of norepinephrine and serotonin.

Physical Conditioning or Deconditioning   Another factor that contributes to the patient's overall pain intensity is physical deconditioning. As pain impedes an individual's normal physical activities of daily living, the body becomes deconditioned, that is, muscles atrophy to various degrees and supporting ligaments weaken. Sometimes deconditioning is the result of other medical conditions, endocrine disorders, or obesity. Unlike normal structures, deconditioned muscles and ligaments are vulnerable and thus unable to handle the stresses and repetitive microtrauma brought about by even the most routine activities. These movements further aggravate the original injury, the end result being additional pain. Depending on the structure involved, body balance may also be impaired because certain muscles, ligaments, and tendons may play an important role in balance and coordination. Thus, in addition to treating the pain generator, supporting structures like muscles and ligaments must likewise be strengthened and healed. This is usually accomplished through a comprehensive physical therapy and rehabilitation program. When this is insufficient, treatments like prolotherapy may supplement the rehabilitation process.

Pain and Related Illnesses or Conditions A third factor that can contribute substantially to the patient's pain intensity is the presence of an illness that is different from the one that is *directly* causing the pain. Some examples are diabetes, with associated neuropathy (which contributes to physical deconditioning); sleep apnea (which in itself leads to depression and weight gain and sleep deprivation, with decreased norepinephrine levels); hypothyroidism and obesity; inflammatory arthritis; smoking; and many others. Treatment of these medical conditions is paramount to the management of chronic pain.

CLASSIFYING BACK PAIN

Physicians use classifications to guide their diagnostic and treatment strategies. As in many medical conditions, classifications are also useful in dealing with painful conditions that affect the spine. Usually experts in the medical community establish criteria for diagnosis (groups of symptoms that define a certain condition) against which the symptoms and signs present in a particular patient are evaluated. Sometimes, a patient may match more than one criterion for the back pain.

Some classifications are based on the causes or specific conditions underlying the mechanisms causing the back pain. One common classification system is as follows (the examples provided are only a few of the most common conditions):

- Mechanical pain
  - Arthritis
  - Degenerated discs
  - Spinal deformities (like scoliosis)
  - Spinal disc herniation (slipped disc)
  - Spinal stenosis (narrowing of the internal spinal canal that contains the spinal cord and its nerves)
  - Spondylolisthesis (an abnormal displacement of one vertebra over another causing damage to the spinal nerves)
  - Fractures
  - Nonspecific muscular or ligamentous strains or sprains
  - Leg length difference
  - Restricted hip motion

- o Misaligned pelvis
- o Muscle or ligament strains
- Inflammatory
  - o Certain inflammatory forms of arthritis (like rheumatoid arthritis, and there are many others)
  - o Infections affecting the bone, discs, or soft tissues
  - o Arachnoiditis—an inflammatory condition that may follow trauma, tumor, infections, bleeding, or administration of various compounds into the spinal fluid. Arachnoiditis can be the cause of neck and back pain; radiating pain in the distribution of the involved nerves; sensory loss in the genital area; occasionally leg weakness or paralysis; and loss of bowel and bladder control.
- Neoplastic
  - o Bone tumors (primary or metastatic)
  - o Spinal tumors
- Metabolic
  - o Osteoporotic vertebral fractures (caused by loss of calcium in the bone). The natural effects of normal aging on the body, in general, and the lower back, in particular, are osteoporosis, or decreased amount of bone. Osteoporosis can lead to bone fractures from a fall or even from the stress of lifting or everyday activities. This can be very painful. Minimally invasive outpatient treatments to seal fractures caused by osteoporosis include injection of a bone like material into the fractured vertebra (vertebroplasty).
  - o Other less common conditions
- Psychosomatic
- Paget's disease (a condition characterized by painful overgrowth of bones)
- Referred pain (pain coming from elsewhere but felt in the spine)
  - o Pelvic/abdominal disease
  - o Prostate cancer

Mike Finds Relief

When Mike saw the orthopedic surgeon for his injured elbow, he was diagnosed with medial epicondylitis and was injected with a steroid. The medial epicondyle is the protrusion at the end of the humerus (upper arm) bone where two tendons and a forearm muscle connect to the bone. It is on the inside of the elbow. Mike experienced no improvement with steroid treatment but decided to give the injury more time to heal. Eight months later, he went to see an upper extremity specialist who again injected him with a steroid. Again, no improvement.

Six months later, Mike was beginning to resign himself to living with a permanent disability. Just touching the palm of his hand to his face or flexing his ring finger and pinkie resulted in pain. Using a screwdriver or a wrench on his three classics cars proved unbearably painful. The only yard work he could manage was to push his lawn mower with his arms fully extended.

In January 2006, Mike was searching for solutions on the Internet and found a link to prolotherapy, a word he had never heard before. Learning more about prolotherapy from a few websites, he decided to give it a try. Mike traveled more than fifty miles each way to my office. He came with some trepidation. Mike was understandably concerned about why so few physicians performed prolotherapy. But realizing that his risk was very small, he decided to give prolotherapy a try. After a few treatments, his condition improved, but he was by no means healed. An MRI confirmed a significant partial tear of the flexor tendon to the medial epicondyle, but I reassured Mike that these types of tears simply take longer than average to repair. Twelve treatments later, Mike was able to return to his usual activities without pain, fear, or reservation. Since then, Mike has returned for treatment of a lateral epicondylitis resulting from a little too much wrenching on his classic cars. Again, he experienced total relief.

The medical community's understanding of pain and all of its dimensions is expanding every day. By understanding your pain better, you will be better prepared to discuss it with your doctor and work together to find the best treatment options for you.

Chapter 3

Taking the First Steps Toward Healing

Jean was approaching retirement age when her left foot began to bother her. As a salesperson in a department store, she had to stand for long periods of time. As the pain worsened, she began to have a hard time standing on her feet; frequently, she would have to sit down and rest her foot. This, of course, interfered with her ability to do her job. She tried some of the simple remedies we would all think of, such as changing shoes and adding supportive inserts. None of these provided relief. Jean eventually sought the help of a foot specialist.

Now that you understand what type of pain you may be experiencing and how pain may be transferred within your body, let's look at some of the first steps you might take in resolving it. The biggest problem with the first steps that we're all accustomed to taking or that we might read about on the Internet is that they might actually do us more harm than good.

RICE, with a Side of Caution

The most basic injuries require equally basic remedies. These types of injuries don't require a trip to the emergency room, and they may not even require a trip to the doctor if you've experienced something similar in the past and know the right steps to take. The most commonly recommended initial treatment for soft tissue injuries is the RICE protocol—rest, ice, compression, and elevation. Various medical advice websites recommend using RICE for many types of injuries, including tendinitis, ligament sprains, strains, and some of the other types of injuries we explored in the previous chapter. But I am raising a giant caution sign at this juncture in our discussion. While RICE may be beneficial in certain types of situations, for many types of soft tissue injuries, it can do *more harm than good*. Here's why.

The purpose of the RICE protocol is to relieve the swelling and pain in the injured area and to give the injury time to heal. All of us have been injured at some point and were probably told to "put ice on it" or "elevate it" or "take an anti-inflammatory medication." If you have a muscle strain and no damage to the surrounding or connected tissues, these steps may work just fine. But if you are dealing with a cartilage, tendon, or ligament injury, RICE could prevent you from healing fully.

As I've described, the tissues around a joint depend on the flow of blood into and around them to deliver the nutrients they need to heal. Inflammation is the result of increased blood flow to the area. Applying ice and/or compression to an injured area seriously decreases the blood flow to the soft tissues and the related cartilage, tendons, and ligaments. Using these treatments for long periods of time is a surefire recipe for chronic pain and reinjury because the soft tissues are unlikely to heal fully or correctly. As you read on, you will learn that inflammation is essential to the healing process, and it is the reason that prolotherapy is so effective.

Now let's look at the rest component of the protocol. Initially, resting an injured body part can prevent you from making the injury worse by using a part of your body that isn't supported by healthy, strong connective tissues. But the basic biology of our joints requires that we move them in order for blood and synovial fluid to flow around and through the various components of the joint, thus furthering the healing process. Resting an injured

> Too much ice, compression, and elevation can actually prevent full or correct healing of injured soft tissues.

joint for long periods of time can cause that joint to freeze. Basically, the joint becomes immovable, and that immobilization can further lead to articular cartilage damage. This occurs because the synovial fluid in the joint is not being refreshed with the nutrients that cartilage needs to remain healthy. That is why it is critical to pair resting the injured joint with gradual, gentle, and regular movement to ensure that the elements of the joint are getting what they need for full and correct healing.

USE OF COMPLEMENTARY TREATMENTS FOR PAIN

According to a study by the National Center for Health Statistics, 37 percent of adults in the United States used some form of complementary or alternative medicine in 2007, many of them to treat pain conditions (Barnes and Bloom, 2008):

- More than 14 million people used complementary therapies for back pain.
- More than 5 million people sought complementary treatment for neck pain.
- About 4.5 million people used complementary therapies for joint pain or stiffness.

Nonsteroidal Anti-inflammatory Agents

You've twisted your ankle. It hurts, and it's starting to swell. What's the first thing you do? Head to the medicine cabinet for some painkillers or anti-inflammatories. Nonsteroidal anti-inflammatory drugs (NSAIDs) help remedy pain by reducing inflammation. NSAIDs are found in almost every grocery store, drugstore, and medicine cabinet in the country. They are frequently used to help reduce fever and to relieve headaches, migraines, muscle pain, menstrual cramps, minor aches, osteoarthritis, sciatica, sprains, strains, dental pain, postoperative pain, and renal colic (pain from kidney stones). Anti-inflammatory drugs account for about 50 percent of all painkillers. Table 3.1 provides a partial list of the NSAIDs available to you either by prescription or over the counter (the kinds for which you don't need a prescription).

NSAIDs are effective for treating the pain associated with very minor injuries, but they should be avoided after an acute injury occurs because they interfere with the healing process. Even though NSAIDs are widely available and are often prescribed for pain resulting from an injury, they should be used with caution. They may be appropriate for chronic inflammatory conditions such as osteoarthritis or rheumatoid arthritis. But more and more research indicates that immediately turning to NSAIDs offers very little benefit, and it may actually limit healing.

For example, in a study published in the *British Medical Journal* in 2002, Kahn et al. found that although many doctors are taught and believe that the first line of treatment for tendinitis should be a course of NSAIDs, more often than not patients actually have tendinosis — not tendinitis — a condition for which the anti-inflammatories do little good. Tendinosis involves tears in the tissue of the tendon, whereas tendinitis is generally thought to be strictly an inflammatory condition. The article also referenced other studies on tendinitis stating:

> A critical review of the role of various anti-inflammatory medications in soft tissue conditions found limited evidence of short-term pain relief and no evidence of their effectiveness in providing even medium term clinical resolution of clearly diagnosed tendon disorders. Laboratory studies have not shown a therapeutic role for these medications.

NSAIDs not only won't help these patients, they also will likely prevent the patient from healing fully and correctly.

Table 3.1: Nonsteroidal Anti-inflammatory Drugs

Brand Name	Generic Name
Advil, Excedrin, Genpril, Haltran, Ibuprin, Ibuprohm, Ibutab, Midrin, Medipren, Midol IB, Motrin, Nuprin, Pamprin-IB, Rufen, Trendar	Ibuprofen
Aleve, Anaprox, Naprosyn	Naproxen sodium
Amigesic, Anaflex 750, Marthritic, mono-Gesic, Salflex, Salsitab, Disalcid	Salsalate
Anacin, Bayer, Bufferin, Ecotrin	Choline salicylate
Ansaid, Froben	Flurbiprofen oral
Apo-Sulin, Clinoril, Novo-Sundac	Sulindac
Aspergum, Genuine Bayer, Bayer Childrens, Bufferin, Easprin, Ecotrin, Empirin, Genprin, Halfprin, Magnaprin, ZORprin	Aspirin
Butazolidin	Phenylbutazone
Cataflam, Voltaren	Diclofenac systemic
DayPro	Oxaprozin
Dolobid	Diflunisal
Feldene, Novo-Pirocam, Nu-Pirox	Piroxicam
Indocin SR, Indocid, Novo Methacin	Indomethacin
Lodine	Etodolac
Meclomen	Meclofenamate sodium
Mobic	Meloxicam
Nalfon	Fenoprofen calcium
Ponstan, Ponstel	Meclofenamic acid
Relafen	Nabumetone
Tolectin	Tolmetin sodium

To understand the pros and cons of NSAIDs, it's helpful to understand exactly how they work. In 1971, it was found that aspirin-like drugs could inhibit the synthesis of a biochemical known as prostaglandin. Prostaglandins are found in nearly all of the body's tissues and organs and have a variety of biochemical and physiologic effects including:

- Constricting or dilating vascular smooth muscle cells,

- Aggregating (clumping together) or disaggregating platelets,
- Regulating the inflammatory process,
- Regulating the movement of calcium,
- Controlling hormonal regulation,
- Controlling cell growth, and
- Regulating blood pressure through the kidneys.

Prostaglandins are produced in cells through the actions of enzymes. By inhibiting the activity of these enzymes, the production of prostaglandins is reduced. The two primary enzymes targeted by NSAIDs are COX-1 and COX-2 (COX stands for cyclooxygenases). Most of the classic NSAIDs work on both COX-1 and COX-2, but newer NSAIDs target merely COX-2. This is generally considered to be an improvement because COX-1 is also responsible for the prostaglandins that support the health of the lining of the inner stomach, which is why NSAIDs can cause ulcers and other stomach problems. COX-2 is primarily responsible for producing prostaglandins that are responsible for inflammation, but the new COX-2 inhibitors have been tied to an increase in the instance or risk of heart attack, thrombosis, or stroke. (Vioxx was pulled from the market because of this.)

Decreasing prostaglandins and therefore decreasing their function can have serious consequences. As mentioned previously, taken regularly for conditions such as arthritis or headaches, NSAIDs can cause ulcers in the stomach or the small intestine. In the small intestine, NSAIDs can cause inflammation and seriously worsen irritable bowel conditions. Allergies to NSAIDs can result in rash, swelling of the face, and difficulty breathing. People with asthma and kidney, heart, or liver impairment should use NSAIDs with caution. In general, NSAIDs should not be used by people who

- Have peptic ulcers or sever acid reflux or indigestion;
- Have a defect of the blood clotting system or who are taking anticoagulants (blood thinners);

- Are pregnant or breastfeeding, except under supervision of a doctor; or

- Have high blood pressure or have had a heart attack or stroke (this involves COX-2 inhibitors specifically).

Before you take an NSAID, or if you have been taking them regularly for any condition, it is important to consult with your physician, especially if you have stomach or bowel problems. No matter what kind of medication you take, you should bring problems to the attention of your physician. As with the RICE protocol, NSAIDs can actually inhibit healing of injured structures, and they are not recommended while you are undergoing prolotherapy, which is explained in detail in chapter 8.

MEAT instead of RICE or NSAIDs

If the RICE protocol and NSAIDs aren't necessarily the best first option, what should you do as a first line of treatment, particularly before you've seen a doctor? Ross A. Hauser, a renowned authority on treating soft tissue injuries and prolotherapy, proposes an alternative to RICE and NSAIDs in his book *Prolo Your Pain Away* (2004). Hauser's protocol goes by the acronym MEAT—movement, exercise, analgesic, and treatment. Let's look at each of these components in a little more detail.

M Is for Movement

It may be hard to imagine using this protocol when you're in pain, but it's possible and beneficial. You can find ways to stay mobile when you are injured. While you may not want to put a lot of pressure on a sprained ankle, you can get up and around on crutches. Moving a joint refreshes the synovial fluid with elements critical to the healing process. If the injury is significant, only passive range of motion exercises should be used—moving the joint gently without weight or stress.

E Is for Exercise

Even if you can't put pressure directly on the injured limb (the ankle in our example), you can do limited, gentle exercises to keep blood flowing well to the site of the injury. You can move the injured joint gently, and apply a little pressure to keep synovial fluid moving around the joint, delivering the critical nutrients that repair and regenerate tissue.

A Is for Analgesic

Analgesics such as acetaminophen (Tylenol) that don't suppress inflammation are a great way to control pain, allowing you to move more without suffering.

The analgesic component of this protocol is particularly important because non-NSAID pain relievers are more likely to support the body's natural healing process. However, some people find that acetaminophen alone doesn't do much to control the pain, particularly if it is acute. Therefore, acetaminophen is combined with other pain relievers, primarily opioids like codeine, and offered in a single tablet or capsule. One example is Tylenol-1, -2, -3, or -4, which are prescription-strength analgesics that contain acetaminophen with different levels of codeine. These types of drugs require a prescription in the United States, so if your pain is acute and you're trying to avoid NSAIDs, you should talk to your doctor about other pain relief options.

T Is for Treatment

With the MEAT protocol, you can treat the injury by seeing a physical therapist, a massage therapist, your family physician, or a doctor who practices regenerative injection therapies, such as prolotherapy. Before you attempt any kind of exercise or rehabilitative treatment, however, you should see a doctor to rule out more severe injuries, such as broken bones, torn tendons, or other injuries that may require more extreme medical treatment.

Your First Trip to the Doctor

Many people live with mild pain without ever seeking help. Is that you? Have you let pain negatively affect your life? Even if your pain is mild, it might not always be so. You should see a doctor as soon as possible if you are in pain.

Pain is a complex issue, and chronic pain can involve contributions from many of your biological systems — musculoskeletal, neurologic, urologic, reproductive, and gastrointestinal. There are no tests that can measure pain, so your doctor must rely on you for a clear description of the pain you feel. You understand the depth and breadth of your pain better than anyone else, even if you don't have a medical degree. What you tell your doctor about your pain is key to diagnosing the underlying problem. Your doctor should ask you for a detailed self-report on the pain. Explain how severe the pain feels in comparison to other pains you've experienced. Unfortunately, some doctors don't fully heed patient self-reports, particularly when patients don't show outward signs of discomfort.

When you visit a doctor about chronic pain, you should also be prepared to provide as much detailed information as possible about the history of the pain, from its onset. If your doctor doesn't seem to be listening, make him. This information should indicate when and how changes in your pain occur, and this is critical in potentially identifying the root cause.

Finally, your doctor should give you a complete physical examination. This is the doctor's opportunity to assess the pain from a professional standpoint. Your physician will also want to determine if there are any psychological or emotional factors that should be taken into consideration. Doctors often consider the effects that emotional responses to the pain — especially those that coincide with chronic pain — have had on a body's ability to heal. Sometimes when other interventions such as traditional medicine or physical therapy have failed, psychological intervention is warranted.

All forms of pain—somatic (acute, chronic) and neuropathic—are serious and should be treated seriously by the physician and the patient. No matter what level of pain you experience, your physician should do everything to help you. Only when the source of your pain has been identified or a viable medical course of action proves useful should your physician quit searching for a healing solution. Physicians must be reminded that pain is a complex issue and varies greatly from patient to patient.

In your attempts to end your pain, you may have taken a variety of over-the-counter remedies, and you might already have seen a physician, likely your family doctor. This is usually the first person people turn to when they are in pain. But when an injury has caused recurring or lasting pain, your primary care physician may quickly exhaust his or her options for helping you heal or for treating your pain. This is when it is critical for you to understand the causes and sources of your pain: It may be up to you to learn how to remedy or control it. When you are in pain, you have to be your own advocate for the best and most appropriate treatment.

> Only when the source of your pain has been identified or a viable medical course of action proves useful should your physician quit searching for a healing solution.

For many patients, complaints of pain to their primary care physician are treated symptomatically. And if the problems are not quickly resolved, the primary care physician becomes a pit stop on the way to various specialists. Julie's experience clearly illustrates the common approach our primary care physicians take toward musculoskeletal injuries—and how it can spin out of control.

Julie was a woman in her mid-forties who had begun experiencing irregular menstrual periods and severe pain in her pelvic area about three years before coming to see me. It seemed reasonable to believe the pain and irregular cycles were connected, although her pain would worsen with movement. When the pain did not resolve with simple analgesics she was sent to a gynecologist who specializes in problems of the female reproductive system. The specialist focused on the irregular periods as the cause of the pain. After numerous tests it was determined that the pain was most likely due to endometriosis. This is a condition in which cells from the lining of the uterus escape into the pelvis, resulting in severe pain, especially during menses. A hysterectomy, including removal of the ovaries, was performed. Unfortunately her pain did not resolve.

Julie returned to her primary care physician and it was decided that perhaps her colon was the cause of the pain. A visit to a gastroenterologist was scheduled and several tests, including a colonoscopy, were performed and nothing specific was found. In such cases it is common to give a nonspecific diagnosis, such as irritable bowel syndrome. Julie was prescribed medications, but they failed to improve her pain.

Again she returned to her primary care physician, complaining that the pain was severe at times, preventing her from doing simple activities. It was beginning to interfere with everything she did. She withdrew from most of her usual social activities. Medications either knocked her out or were ineffective. Several times the pain became so severe that she went directly to the emergency room, where she was given more ineffective medications.

She had been in pain for more than a year when her doctor referred her to a urologist (a doctor who specializes in conditions of the bladder and urinary tract). After several tests, including a cystoscopy, nothing specific was found and she was treated for another nonspecific condition known as interstitial cystitis. However, the medications commonly given for this condition did nothing for her pain and she discontinued the medications on her own.

Still seeking a solution she returned again to her primary care physician. Since there were no more organs in the area to examine, her physician felt that perhaps the pain was secondary to an injury to her lower abdominal wall above her pelvic area. She was therefore sent to a general surgeon who specialized in repairs of a herniated abdominal wall. After an exam and tests it was decided that the cause of the pain was a tear in the abdominal wall above her pelvic area. Julie underwent surgery to repair the presumed tear. But as before, after the procedure, her original pain did not go away. Worse yet, she now began to experience a jabbing pain with certain movements in addition to her original pain.

After three years of constant pain and ineffective treatments, Julie was desperate. She and her husband had been patients of mine before they had moved a few years before, and she returned to me for help. When she came into my office and told me of her three-year battle and the tests and procedures she had endured, I was shocked. Her life was very limited and sad. As I listened to the long story of her ordeal and took a medical history, I noticed she had lost a lot of weight. Complementing her on her accomplishment I asked her how she did it. Julie explained that before she got hurt she was exercising regularly with Pilates. I didn't know much about Pilates but I have seen ads depicting slender women arched on their backs over a large rubber ball. With that image in mind it hit me. I immediately asked Julie to lie down on the examining table. I palpated along her pubis, where her abdominal wall joins, and she nearly jumped off the table. "Well there's the problem!" I exclaimed. "Didn't any of the physicians examine you thoroughly?" Julie replied that she had told them that the pain was just above her pubic bone. But I had just discovered, very simply, that Julie's pain was the result of a stretched tendon where the rectus abdominal muscle attaches to the pubic bone.

Happily, after several prolotherapy treatments Julie's pain resolved. She has since returned to a more active lifestyle. The last I heard, she was enjoying a cruise.

How such a seemingly obvious problem could be missed reveals a problem with our healthcare system: very few primary care physicians are ever trained sufficiently in soft tissue injuries. And specialists are focused on their own areas of expertise. The insurance companies do not pay them to think beyond their specialty.

Mike is another patient of mine whose case is similar to Julie's in some ways. He came to my office in early 2008 after returning from Iraq on a short leave. Mike came in complaining of lower abdominal pain and was afraid he might have a hernia. The pain came and went especially with lifting. When I was reviewing his history, he told me he had gone to Iraq at the end of 2007 as a contracted electrician to earn extra money for his family. During his time off he would exercise. Mike was impressed with the physique of some of the young military guys and was resolved to return to his family with a "six pack." He began doing strenuous sit-ups and abdominal crunches. Just like Julie, his pain was along the top of his pubis. He received a cortisone injection along the attachment of the rectus abdominal muscle and within a few days his pain resolved. In Mike's case the pain was purely inflammatory in nature without an associated tear, which I could determine by the fact that the pain resolved without recurrence, even with strenuous activity. If Mike had seen another physician, he might have undergone the same battery of tests and specialists that Julie had.

Who to See: A Specialist or a Generalist

When patients come to see me, it is often after they have already seen an orthopedic or pain medicine physician. As a family physician, I call on such specialists every day to help me manage my patients' conditions. Starting your care with a specialist, however, is not always the best way to begin treatment for soft tissue injuries that result in pain, even chronic pain.

Orthopedic and neurosurgeons are extremely well trained and are often consulted in cases of chronic pain. However, soft tissue injuries can often masquerade as a neurological problem. I always remind people that if a woman over fifty were to go to the emergency room complaining of left arm pain, she would not have her arm examined. Instead, an EKG and cardiac enzyme test would be performed to rule out an acute heart attack. The heart, which is a muscle, can refer pain to the chest, neck, jaw, or left arm. Tendons and ligaments can refer pain as well. Not every radiating pain is nerve pain. Unfortunately, if you know very little about soft tissue injuries you may misinterpret the chronic pain as a sign of the need for surgery. But the collateral damage from surgery is often unacceptable, as I'll discuss in chapter 9.

The best approach to diagnosing and treating most soft tissue injuries and the pain that can accompany them is a multifaceted treatment approach. Resolution of pain, particularly chronic pain, often requires peeling away the various causes. The initial cause of pain can result in a domino effect, affecting one body part and then another and then another. Returning to a pain-free condition requires more than merely treating the initial cause of the pain. It is necessary to address all the systems involved in the domino effect. Generalists are well equipped to do just that because they are accustomed to addressing a variety of interacting disease processes. Specialists (perhaps with the exception of some pain medicine physicians, as discussed in the next paragraph) often focus on only one component of the pain, usually those areas in which they are skilled. This focus lacks objectivity. And by seeing a specialist, you may skip over simpler treatment options. I tell my patients it is best to start with the simpler treatments and then move to the more complex—in other words, to move from the less risky to the more risky.

While you may not want to immediately see a specialist in terms of a neurologist or an orthopedic surgeon, if you are experiencing chronic pain, you may need to consider seeing an interventional pain medicine physician. Pain medicine is a growing multidisciplinary specialty area that primarily deals with the causes and treatments of the conditions causing chronic pain. Pain physicians use minimally invasive techniques to diagnose and treat an array of painful conditions. In addition to the role in discovering the source of a patient's primary pain, he or she will assist coordinating a multidisciplinary approach for the treatment, which will include your primary care doctor.

A Simple Case: Seeking the Source of Pain

In his book, *How Doctors Think* (2008), Jerome Groopman, MD, described his ordeal with the medical system after experiencing an injury to his right wrist. It initially began with twinges in both wrists from many hours of "banging clumsily" on his computer. This pain resolved with rest until he injured his right wrist while swimming (another swimmer struck his wrist during a downward stroke). Ice temporarily improved the pain until Dr. Groopman injured his wrist again—this time when using it to stop an elevator door. The straw that broke the camel's back occurred while he was trying to remove the lid from a fruit juice bottle and experienced severe pain at the base of his thumb. This appeared to be a classic case of a soft tissue injury. So long as Dr. Groopman avoided using his wrist, he would have temporary relief. Just as Dr. Groopman described, pain that accompanies certain positions or particular uses can often signal ligamental instability. Joint instability may result in chronic joint inflammation and swelling.

Dr. Groopman decided to see a well-known hand surgeon. After many weeks of splinting, then not splinting, and an MRI that showed nothing, the doctor suggested surgery. But Dr. Groopman didn't buy into the diagnosis, so he refused surgery, fearing that it would do more harm than good. He then consulted another doctor, who felt that several surgeries would be necessary to correct the problem. That doctor predicted it would take one to two years before Dr. Groopman would recover, assuming that all went well. Dr. Groopman went to another famed hand surgeon, who also could not offer a plausible diagnosis— and also recommended surgery.

Finally, Dr. Groopman saw a fourth doctor, who determined that a lax, or partially torn, ligament in his wrist was the cause of the pain. The instability resulted in friction—a rubbing of the bones—thereby triggering a chronic inflammatory state. This seemed to be the correct diagnosis. Dr. Groopman underwent surgery in which he used a recently developed synthetic bone material for grafting to repair the torn ligament and five months of rehabilitation, after which he felt that his wrist was 80 percent better. Although he was satisfied with the results, he was left with some discomfort and limitation. In my experience, it's likely that the pain to his right wrist will eventually worsen over time.

Dr. Groopman has several advantages over most of my own patients. As a physician himself, he was able to discern the inaccuracies of the earlier diagnoses and proposed treatments. He was also able to afford consultations with many different medical experts. But did Dr. Groopman really get the best treatment despite his huge advantages? I think not. I have treated people with simple wrists sprains, most resolving totally. Was going straight to a hand specialist really necessary? We will never know if a few prolotherapy treatments or platelet-rich plasma injections (discussed in chapter 7) would have resolved his injury, but this is where he should have started. Unfortunately, he did not seek this option. In this respect, some of my patients have an advantage over Dr. Groopman. By having a healthy skepticism and fear of surgery, they discovered the option of prolotherapy. When Dr. Groopman was finally given the correct diagnosis of ligamental laxity, he did not consider that another possible treatment option to surgery existed, nor was he given the option of regenerative injection therapies.

Although you may not want to immediately see a specialist such as a neurologist or an orthopedic surgeon, if you are experiencing chronic pain, you may need to consider seeing an interventional pain management physician.

Be an Advocate for Your Healing

Without the Internet, many patients would be stuck with intractable symptoms that make life almost intolerable. One such patient was Tim, who began to experience tingling in the back of his neck two years before coming to see me. The feeling was not painful but was very noticeable during different times of the day. Tim did notice that the symptoms occurred particularly after working hours on the computer. After months of intermittent tingling, Tim began to wake in the morning with numbness to the lower left side of his cheek and began to experience neck pain. Before long the numbness and tingling spread to both sides of his face. This was soon followed by a bout of dizziness. Tim told coworkers that he felt off balance. When the pain spread to the area behind his eyes and over his sinuses, Tim thought perhaps he had a sinus infection, although he thought it odd that he had no symptoms of congestion or fever. Nonetheless, Tim tried over the counter treatments for sinusitis.

About seven months after his symptoms began he awoke with such severe dizziness that he decided to go to a local emergency room. After he described all his symptoms, the ER physician diagnosed him with sinusitis and prescribed a ten-day course of antibiotics. Following up with his family physician, Tim continued to complain of dizziness and an anti-dizziness medicine, Antivert, was prescribed.

Weeks went by and Tim was still experiencing dizziness. Then he began to notice episodes of heart palpitations. When a battery of tests done by his doctor came back normal he was sent to a cardiologist. The cardiologist did verify the palpitations on a heart monitor but was unable to explain all the other symptoms. Tim was assured that the palpitations did not appear to be life threatening.

Desperate for immediate relief from his symptoms, particularly the dizziness that was making it difficult for him to function, Tim returned to his family physician. This time he was given a small patch to place behind his ear, a treatment commonly used to prevent seasickness. Again, nothing. Tim was then sent to an ear, nose, and throat specialist. The ENT physician ordered a CT scan of the sinuses, which came back normal. Nonetheless a diagnosis of chronic sinusitis was made. Again, the treatment made no difference in Tim's symptoms.

One morning Tim awoke with a sharp pain in his chest. After he was admitted to the hospital, numerous tests were run, including a CT scan of his chest and abdomen, EKG, blood work, and chest x-rays. Tim was discharged the next morning when everything came back normal.

After nearly a year with these symptoms, Tim decided to try acupuncture, but found no relief. A friend suggested he try a doctor of internal medicine. The new doctor was also convinced his symptoms were sinus related, and Tim was given another trial of antibiotics. Eventually, he was referred out for another ENT opinion with no solution found.

Researching his condition online, Tim began to fear that perhaps he had an undiagnosed neurological disorder. The neurologist ordered an MRI of the brain and neck. Again nothing.

Having suffered for more than two years, Tim refused to accept that he would have to endure a limited life and he returned to the Internet. Entering 7 or 8 of his main symptoms, Tim pulled up information about Barre-Lieou syndrome, which is characterized by a wide range of symptoms including the ones he was experiencing. The cause of Barre-Lieou syndrome is instability of the cervical vertebral bodies due to ligament laxity. It is thought that this instability leads to the malfunction of the posterior cervical sympathetic nervous system, which is found near the cervical vertebrae. I had seen these symptoms many times and treated them successfully as part of whiplash injuries, but had never diagnosed the condition in someone who hadn't experienced any trauma. I found in my research that ligament laxity may occur over a long period of time due to poor posture with the head in a forward position. Tim's work for long hours in front of a computer probably explains the cause.

Treating Tim's ligaments along the cervical spine and along the muscle attachments to the base of the skull resolved his symptoms. Unfortunately, there are no tests to diagnose this condition. Had Tim seen me at the very beginning of his condition, I may have treated him initially in a similar manner as the other physicians and eventually referred him to specialists. Only when more common conditions are ruled out would I have considered Barre-Lieou. In this particular case it helped that Tim was able to point me in the right direction and was versed in prolotherapy.

Whether you're experiencing chronic or acute pain, prolotherapy may be the solution you have been waiting days, weeks, months, or possibly years to receive. Restoring a patient's function sufficiently so that he or she can provide for the family — pride intact — or allowing an athlete to fulfill dreams or preventing a patient from making a decision that might result in lifelong chronic pain is the real advantage of prolotherapy. With prolotherapy many patients have resolved their discomfort from repetitive activity or one unfortunate accident. Remember Jean from the beginning of the chapter?

The specialist Jean saw about her foot pain, which was diagnosed as plantar fasciitis, gave her a steroid injection. She experienced excellent but temporary relief. Repeating the injection did not resolve the tenderness. By the time Jean came to see me, I could hardly touch her heel without making her scream. Jean was unable to take long walks, as she once had, and had consequently gained weight. The increased weight placed still more stress on the painful tendon in her heel, making walking even more difficult. Surgery was an option she wanted to avoid, and she was willing to give prolotherapy a try. After only nine treatments, Jean was back to walking three miles a day as part of her regular exercise program and could stand for prolonged periods without pain.

Like Jean and Tim, relief from your pain may be just an office visit away.

Chapter 4

Tests: What Do They Really Show?

Jeff was an inspector at a local chemical plant where he did repetitive bending and lifting. Twenty years ago, while lifting the tools he used on a daily basis, he felt a sharp pain in his lower back. So severe was the pain that it immediately brought him to his knees. Weeks went by, and with the use of over-the-counter medication, the pain slowly disappeared. Jeff seemed to have recovered. Afterward, he would suffer bouts of low back pain several times a year, but it was never severe and the cause was not identifiable. Five years later, however, the low back pain returned, and it became severe. Instead of random instances of pain, it was a constant companion and was at times unbearable. Jeff again battled the pain with medication, but it began to interfere with Jeff's work and family activities. Based on an abnormal MRI and, at the advice of a surgeon, Jeff had two discs from his lower back removed. Then the hell really began. Weeks later, when recovery should have been complete, the pain was still very much a part of his everyday life, much to Jeff's disappointment. Another MRI revealed that his persistent pain was presumably due to two more abnormal discs. After these were removed in a second surgery, the pain became even worse.

Many of us place too much faith in medical tests and know too little about them. When or if you were told to have an MRI, would you know why? Do you know what an MRI is, what it reveals, or why a doctor would choose an MRI over another test? Most people don't know the difference between X-rays, CT scans, or MRIs. What are the consequences of not understanding these tests? You rely heavily on their results without the knowledge of what the results actually mean or whether the results of any one of these tests is the truest factor in determining treatment options. This combination may make you vulnerable to making poor health care decisions and possibly incurring more pain and expense.

Take a moment to reflect on this scenario: The surgeon comes in, introduces herself, and sits with you for ten minutes to determine whether surgery is necessary. The decision might be made on the basis of an X-ray or an MRI, which has confirmed that there is an injury. There is no discussion about possible soft tissue damage, that is, damage to neighboring tendons, ligaments, or muscles. Although complete tears of ligaments and tendons are obvious and usually do require surgery, incomplete or microscopic tears are much less obvious but equally as important to your recovery. If these don't show up on the test, your doctor may never talk to you about how to help them heal. And if the test is not accurate and you actually have just a sprain, the outcome of surgery could be worse than your current condition. Undergoing surgery to repair sprained ligaments is like using a sledgehammer to drive in a nail. It will work, but at a great cost—physically, financially, and possibly mentally. The resulting damage can be both unacceptable and irreversible. Situations like this are avoidable for the educated patient. Understanding the different tests that you are asked to undergo may be the first step toward finding a solution to the pain you are in and ensuring that you are on the right path to proper and complete healing.

X-Rays

X-rays are the most common test used to determine whether a bone has been injured or fractured. Using electromagnetic radiation, an X-ray machine takes a photograph, of sorts, of the injured area (see figures 4.1 and 4.2 on the next pages). The resulting image is of dense masses within the body, mainly bones, and is used to identify broken bones or hairline fractures. In some cases, such as pneumonia, X-rays can also be used to locate masses in the lungs or other soft tissue organs. Because X-rays cannot detect many injuries within soft tissue surrounding bones, most doctors rely on CT scans or MRIs to locate the source of soft tissue pain, particularly after they've ruled out bone injury based on an X-ray.

If you are like most people, you have probably had an X-ray taken at some point in your life, so you know that the procedure is quick and easy, which is a definite advantage. You lie down or stand in front of a large box that contains film. A technician moves the X-ray machine over or in front of you, directs it at the injury, and ZAP, he takes the X-ray. The film is then developed and analyzed.

But X-rays can be discouraging when you are in pain. If you see your doctor with a complaint of wrist pain, an X-ray may be in order to help diagnose the problem. When the X-ray results show no break or dislocation, you may begin to question the cause of the pain and whether there is any hope for relief. This is the most serious limitation of X-rays. They are unable to detect all types of injuries, leaving many patients without answers and solutions for their pain. So the next step is typically a CT scan or MRI.

Figure 4.1: X-ray of the Knee

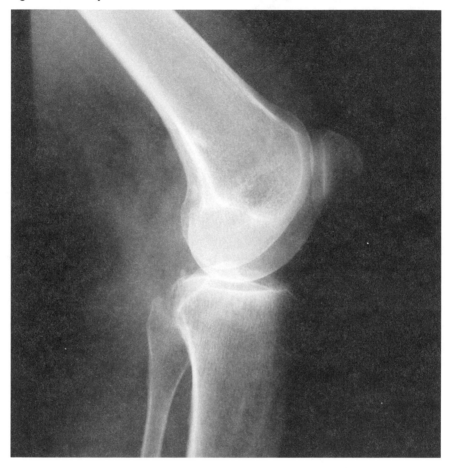

CT Scan

Computerized tomography (CT) scans (also called CAT scans for com-
puted axial tomography) reveal a more complete diagnosis of an injury
by taking multiple X-ray images from different angles around a single
axis point, the point of injury. By combining many two-dimensional
images, a CT scan creates a three-dimensional image of the inside of
the body that can show the full extent of an injury that a simple X-ray
cannot identify (see figure 4.3). This allows for a far more accurate

Figure 4.2: X-ray of the Shoulder

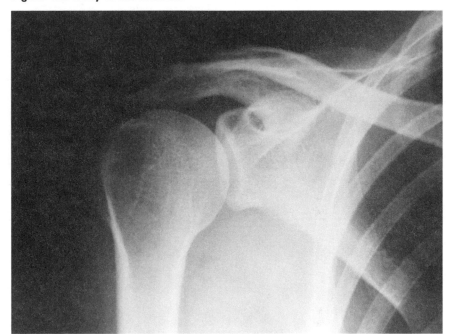

diagnosis of certain types of injuries and diseases or disorders. There are many different types of CT scans, and the type used may depend on what part of the body or what condition is being tested. CT scans can be used to identify masses in organs, embolisms, blood flow and digestive flow problems, and many other issues. When it comes to joint or back injuries, CT scans are not as effective as MRI scans (which are discussed in the next section) in identifying soft tissue injuries around bones. CT scans are helpful, however, in creating images of complex fractures and ligament tears.

If you are getting a CT scan for a joint injury, you will be asked to lie on a long table. The table will move you through an opening in the middle of a large machine, and you will need to remain very still. The scan will take a bit of time because many images are being taken. The table might move forward or backward slightly as the machine repositions you to capture images from more angles.

Figure 4.3: CT Scan of an Injured Knee

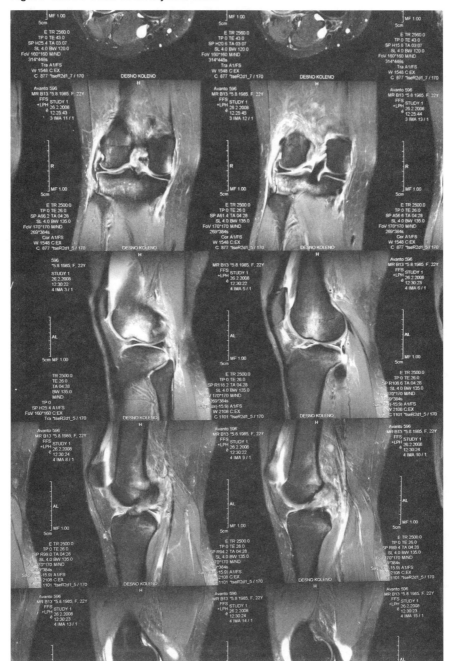

Although CT scans can be very informative, they are also relatively expensive, so doctors usually reserve this particular test for heart or lung problems or to locate and diagnose cancer.

MRI

For injuries to joints or backs, the most often used — and the most often misunderstood — test is the magnetic resonance imaging (MRI) test. This incredible piece of technology is used to evaluate the anatomy of a particular body structure. Though similar in many ways to a CT scan, the MRI shows a greater contrast in the soft tissue areas of the body; consequently, it is much better at revealing damage to these tissues. Multiple cross-sectional images of the injured area are taken, revealing damage to bones as well as soft tissues (see figures 4.4 and 4.5). MRIs are particularly helpful with joint and back injuries because they show not only the bones and joints clearly but also the tendons, ligaments, and muscles. Another benefit of MRIs is that they are safer overall than CT scans because they don't use X-rays, which produce ionizing radiation.

One problem with MRIs is that they can be uncomfortable. An MRI machine looks like a very thick doughnut. When you undergo an MRI, you lie on a narrow table that moves you into the MRI machine. The opening is narrow, and you are fully enclosed by the machine. For people who experience claustrophobia, an MRI can be a difficult procedure to endure. But the resulting images are extremely useful for determining the next course of action to promote healing. Another problem with MRIs is that they are very costly, much more so than CT scans are, so doctors may be reluctant to order them unless your injury seems severe or your pain is chronic and intense enough to warrant them.

Unfortunately, even though they are often helpful, MRI results can be misinterpreted or misleading. There have been many cases when surgery was recommended for injuries such as disc herniation

Figure 4.4: MRI Scan of a Foot

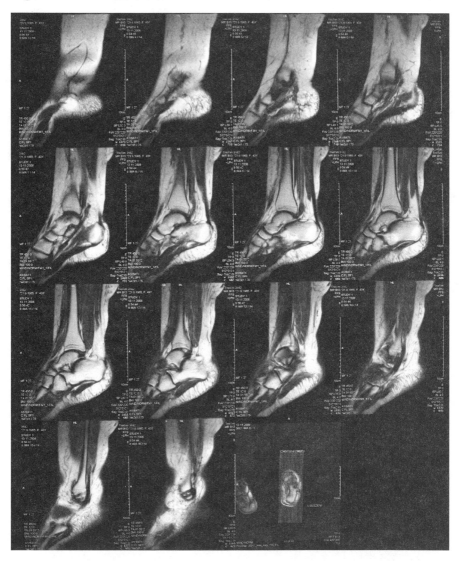

based solely on MRI results and because a patient's back pain had not resolved with physical therapy and medicine. But jumping to the surgery option is not always the best course of action (remember Freddie from the introduction). The tests that are relied on to indicate surgery cannot predict the benefits from that surgery.

Figure 4.5: MRI Scan of the Cervical Spine

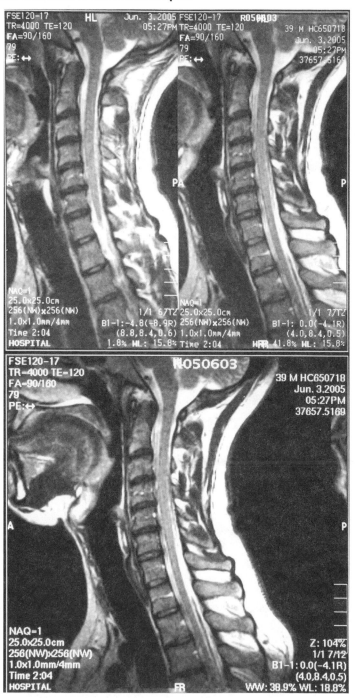

Ultrasounds

Ultrasounds are increasingly being used to identify soft tissue injuries. Ultrasounds (also called sonograms) work by bouncing high-frequency sound waves off of tissues in the body. The denser the tissue, the more echogenic it is, that is, the better it is at reflecting the sound waves. Ligaments and tendons can be viewed with ultrasound technology, and injuries or abnormalities to those tissues may be clear. Think of the amazing three-dimensional scans you've seen in science magazines or books of babies in utero. Now imagine that technology applied to the tissues in your shoulder or your spine.

Ultrasounds generally cost less than CTs and MRIs, although ultrasounds may not be as good at detecting some types of soft tissue injuries. Also, the denser the tissue, the more the ultrasound will show only the outward shape of the structure and may not reveal problems deeper within a joint. Nevertheless, ultrasounds are proving useful in guiding certain types of therapies—particularly regenerative injection therapies like prolotherapy—to the exact spot of injury.

Dynamic Radiographic Computerized Analysis

Although the various tests just described can show some aspects of soft tissue injury, few can show one of the main culprits of back pain—ligament laxity, more commonly known as loose ligaments. This laxity is important to diagnose because it could lead to more serious soft tissue damage and injury. Dynamic radiographic computerized analysis is one method that can be used to diagnose ligament laxity. It involves taking a series of X-rays while the body or body part is in different positions, such as flexion, extension, and neutral, and marking specific points on the vertebral bodies in the images. Then an objective computer analysis can determine whether the vertebral body has slipped out of its normal alignment. Hypermobility, or the ability to stretch joints farther than normal, provides evidence of weakened, injured ligaments. This particular testing method can also be used to record the neck or back in motion and allows the physician to see the abnormal movement associated with ligament laxity. Test results from dynamic radiographic computerized analysis support the use of prolotherapy as a treatment. It would be nearly impossible to accurately diagnose loose ligaments with just an MRI or an X-ray.

What You See Is Not Necessarily What You Have

Patients frequently bring in MRI results that were ordered by another physician and ask how I can treat their bulging disc or herniated disc. When I ask my patients what those terms mean, they typically do not know. What the patients do know, however, is that the MRI is abnormal, which they assume explains their back pain (acute or chronic). It is often the case that there is an abnormality, *but abnormalities are not always the source of pain.* If you are about to undergo (or have undergone) an MRI, it's important for you to be familiar with some of the terms you may see.

TERMS YOU MIGHT SEE ON AN MRI REPORT

- *Spondylosis* is a nonspecific term that refers to any degenerative lesion of the spine, similar to arthritis.
- *Facet arthropathy* is a condition of arthritic changes to the facet joint, where the vertebrae connect to one another.
- *Degenerative disc disease* is related to the progressive worsening of the physical characteristics of the discs in the spine and is commonly associated with the normal aging process.
- *Degenerative disease of the facet joints* is a progressive worsening of the physical characteristics of the facet joint, also commonly associated with the normal aging process.
- *Bulged or protruded discs* are small herniations that generally do not involve spinal or nerve compression.

- *Herniated disc* describes large disc herniations that can be seen on an MRI, confirming spinal or nerve compression.
- *Anterolisthesis* refers to the movement of the vertebral bodies forward, out of normal alignment.
- *Retrolisthesis* refers to the movement of the vertebral bodies backward, out of normal alignment.
- *Osteophyte* is a bony outgrowth from the vertebral body, possibly resulting from an old calcified injury.
- *Spinal stenosis* indicates a narrowing of the spinal canal, usually from arthritic changes that may constrict the spinal column.
- *Foraminal stenosis* indicates a narrowing of the foramen (the opening between vertebrae through which nerves exit the spine and extend to other parts of the body) usually as a result of arthritic changes that may constrict the nerve as it leaves the spinal column.

Assuming that a patient has any of these abnormalities, how likely is it that they account for the pain they may be experiencing? In one study, sixty-seven volunteers with no low back pain were given a free MRI of the lumbar spine (Boden et al., 1990). Among the volunteers older than sixty years of age, the MRI found that 37 percent had herniated discs and 21 percent had evidence of spinal stenosis. Yet, these men and women had no complaints of back pain. The researchers also found that 35 percent of the volunteers who were between twenty and thirty-nine years of age had evidence of degenerative disc disease, yet they also had no pain whatsoever. In another study, Jensen and her colleagues (1994) identified disc bulges in the MRIs of 52 percent of their ninety-eight volunteers who reported no low back pain. In addition, the MRIs identified that 14 percent of the volunteers had degenerative disc disease of the facet joints, 8 percent had spondylosis, 7 percent had spondylolisthesis, and 7 percent had spinal stenosis. Despite the diagnoses, these volunteers had no back pain. Yet, surgery might have been recommended for them had they presented with back pain.

In another study, sixty volunteers with no complaints of back pain underwent an MRI scan (Weishaupt et al., 1998). Of these, 18 percent had evidence of severe disc herniation, and 2 percent had severe nerve root compression. In this study, patients who had no symptoms were scanned, as were those at high risk of back problems because of the type of work they did, such as construction workers or roadwork crew members. Researchers found that the rate of false positives was high among those who did frequent bending, twisting, heavy lifting, and working with vibration equipment (such as riveters). The results further showed that the MRIs of 76 percent of the asymptomatic subjects — that is, patients with no symptoms — had a least one herniated disc, 13 percent of which were severe! Seventeen percent of the pain-free subjects had evidence of minor root compression and 4 percent had evidence of severe root compression.

If these so-called high-risk individuals with asymptomatic herniated discs had injured themselves during the course of their heavy work and failed to improve with conservative treatment consisting of physical therapy and chiropractic manipulation, many would have been considered good candidates for surgery. And most of those would have had the recommended surgery. If you hurt your back from lifting heavy objects, sprain a tendon or a ligament, and have an attendant severe muscle spasm, one thing is sure: Operating on an asymptomatic disc only makes things worse. If you then become disabled, the monetary and human costs go through the roof.

Patients frequently become concerned when they learn that their MRI has identified degenerative disc disease, and rightly so. Any indication of disease in your body should trigger your concern. But this is not a cause for panic. Nearly 50 percent of middle-aged individuals (forty to fifty-

> Nearly 50 percent of middle-aged individuals who have no back pain at all have evidence of degenerative disc disease.

nine years old) who have no back pain at all have evidence of degenerative disc disease. If you find this in your report, it does not necessarily explain your pain. This is especially true for persons older than sixty whose job includes some type of physical labor. Almost 19 percent of normal fourteen-year-olds without back pain had evidence of degenerative disc disease verified by an MRI (Heck et al., 2007). So, even though the MRI results would have been interpreted to indicate a need for surgery, or at least physical therapy, these teenagers experienced no back pain. Once again, we caution that a test, be it an MRI, a CT scan, or an X-ray, should not be the single indicator of whether surgery is the solution.

These and many other studies clearly show that abnormalities in discs or vertebrae alone do not automatically mean corresponding back or leg pain. Unfortunately, however, that exact assumption is what physicians most quickly identify through tests like MRIs. But before an MRI leads a patient straight to the operating table, all parties involved should consider the possibility of soft tissue injury.

Remember Jeff, the chemical plant inspector introduced at the beginning of the chapter? Based on MRIs, he underwent two surgeries to remove discs thought to be the cause of his pain. Still later, he was forced to undergo a third surgery, a fusion of the vertebrae in his lumbar spine, or low back, using titanium rods and screws. According to Jeff, his surgeon said that this surgery was guaranteed to relieve the pain. It didn't. To add insult to this unrelenting injury, Jeff incurred a huge hospital bill — more than $125,000.

Out of desperation, Jeff agreed to yet another surgery to remove those same rods and screws. They had begun to press on nerves in his back, which was making an aggravating pain virtually intolerable. The list of unsuccessful remedies for Jeff grew longer: a morphine pump, nerve stimulators, narcotic strength medication. Yet, the pain continued.

Jeff came to my office distraught. Sobbing, he relayed his story. Had he known he would end up like this, he never would have allowed the surgeons to operate on his back. His pain now was more than physical. Almost twenty years of constant back pain, and every type of solution having failed him, this injury had affected his emotional health as well as his financial and relational health. He hadn't had sex with his wife in more than five years, a factor that was instrumental in their divorce. Jeff was a deacon in a church, but he had not been able to attend owing to his chronic pain. His last place of comfort and refuge had been denied him. Every night, he said, he prayed that God would take him in his sleep. But every morning he woke up, still in pain. Eight years after that first surgery, Jeff was a fifty-seven-year-old man who depended on his elderly mother to take care of him on a day-to-day basis.

I was very sad after hearing Jeff's story, but I was also angry with the physicians who had put him in this position. Would Jeff's life have been different had the physicians considered that the results of the MRIs, while showing abnormalities, might not be revealing the true cause of his pain? Had those MRI tests really shown the problem or just a portion of it? Was there a soft tissue injury that was left unidentified? Prolotherapy may have changed the course of Jeff's life. And I think about that every time a new patient comes through the door.

After my conversations with Jeff (and Freddie, the soccer coach I mentioned in the introduction), I never looked at an MRI in quite the same way again. Thinking also of those patients with indicative MRIs but no pain, I wondered, if one of those individuals were to eventually hurt her back badly enough to require evaluation by an MRI, would the asymptomatic herniated disc lead to an unnecessary surgery? An unnecessary surgery could result in a worsening of her pain and a permanent disability. An inappropriate surgery could result in lifelong pain, an inability to work, and severe depression.

If you look at the results of the various studies that have been conducted (some of which I mentioned previously), you can safely say that more than half of all individuals older than forty years of age have abnormal MRIs. This should not be surprising. As someone well over that age, I can relate. I commonly explain to my patients that my face is now no longer *normal* as I knew normal when I was younger. I have some white hair, somewhat wrinkled skin, and little bumps I did not have when I was twenty. Is what are commonly referred to as abnormal bulges, arthritic changes, and loss of disc height really that abnormal for someone who has been active for more than forty years? I think not. Yet, this common age-related change is often given as a reason for surgery. Unfortunately, if you are in a lot of pain and a very well-educated surgeon tells you that one of these common abnormalities is the cause of your pain, you are apt to agree.

Predicting Future Problems

Not long ago, many companies routinely required that all their prospective employees have a lumbar X-ray, especially those who would engage in physical labor and had a history of frequent back injury claims. This practice has generally been abandoned, though, because it has proven worthless in predicting future claims. Because most back injuries result from the physical rigors of the job, combined with a poor lifting technique and the poor condition of the employee, any previous back X-ray is not a strong factor in predicting the future possibility of injury. None of these causative factors is measured by an X-ray. Even MRIs cannot predict future back injury. MRIs, CT scans, and X-rays are rarely able to demonstrate soft tissue injuries that are present, much less ones that have yet to happen.

Overreliance on Tests

In the managed-care environment, hospitals and private medical practices attempt to avoid unnecessary testing because of lawsuit-happy patients who believe they have received inadequate or improper treatment. However, doctors frequently order tests to be conducted and use the results as proof of medical conditions or a lack thereof. The problem is not related so much to the unwarranted ordering of tests as to an overreliance on them to justify the need for treatment and/or surgery. As you have seen, this practice can lead to unnecessary surgeries and poor treatment outcomes.

Tests are merely one view of the injury, a look at the situation from only one perspective. To be able to fully diagnose an injury, particularly a soft tissue injury, it is wise to have more than one assessment tool. The technology used in modern science, and in creating the tests described in this chapter, is truly phenomenal, and much has been gained from technological invention. However, to rely on tests as the sole factor in deciding whether to have surgery is a costly and possibly painful mistake. Having a working knowledge of the types of tests given by doctors, as well as understanding their restrictions, helps you, as the patient, see the true, though limited, value of X-rays, CT scans, and MRIs. Test results should be combined with professional medical evaluation as well as patient knowledge to determine what steps you should take to begin the recovery process.

Chapter 5

Options for Treating Pain

Nancy was in a car accident in 1983. Minimally injured, she recovered from the back pain caused by the accident and returned to life as normal. But in 1990, Nancy was in a car that was involved in a head-on collision at an intersection. Unbelievably, a year later her car was rear-ended by another vehicle. After each accident, her level of back pain increased significantly. An MRI revealed that she had two degenerated discs in the lumbar area and three in the cervical area.

The pain from the combined injuries was almost impossible for Nancy to bear. Even short walks were out of the question. Her life consisted of sitting in a recliner. She had learned to let the housework go undone. She could not do the crafts she so enjoyed because her hands shook as she worked and she could not bend her neck to look down. Cooking holiday meals was a thing of the past.

Members of her family begged Nancy to use her computer so they could communicate with her by email. She attempted to sit at the computer for short periods of time, but the pain was always so severe that she was unable to stay there for long. She became increasingly isolated. There was no comfort—sitting still was painful and walking was virtually impossible. In the early summer of 2003, she and her husband decided to attempt a slow stroll through EPCOT in Orlando. It was during that trip that she remarked to her husband that her next trip to Disney World would have to be in a wheelchair. She was experiencing shooting pains down her legs from the degenerated discs in her lower back.

Have you suffered in some of the same ways Nancy has? If so, how did you feel about your future? As we've already discussed, no matter how long you've had your pain, and no matter whether it is new or chronic, a helpful mind-set for you to adopt is to think of the origin of the pain and to focus on the injury. If you are injured, there is hope for recovery and an end to the pain.

Once you've decided to do something about your pain, the next step is to explore all of your treatment options. Every doctor's experiences are different, and therefore every doctor's plan for your treatment might be different in small or even large ways. And while I believe that it's critical for anybody in pain to address the underlying problem to achieve lasting relief, I also recognize that you probably bought this book because you are currently in pain and are seeking relief right away. So, in this chapter I'm going to outline your pain relief options. Some of them are noninvasive, preliminary treatments for immediate pain relief, and some are invasive, extreme treatments that should be used only in the most extreme situations.

Pain Medications

For most people who are injured and for those who have been suffering for some time, the first thought in terms of treatment is getting rid of the pain. Therefore, even though pain medications won't generally resolve an injury, they are nonetheless a treatment option that needs to be carefully examined. In chapter 3, I discussed NSAIDs and why they may not be your best first option; yet for some people, resolving the pain might never require more than an analgesic like Tylenol during the healing process. But many other types of pain medications may be recommended or prescribed when someone has an injury.

After the third car accident, Nancy's orthopedic surgeon put her on a full-time regimen of NSAIDs, including COX-2 inhibitors, and muscle relaxants. Those drugs were helpful in getting the pain to a manageable level. Although she still could do very little, she some-how managed to get through each day. The side effects, however, were difficult to live with. She couldn't read a book because the medicines made her so sleepy, she couldn't get through more than a page. Also, over time, the NSAIDs took a toll on her body. Her stomach hurt non-stop and her blood pressure was high. NSAIDs were obviously not the solution that Nancy was looking for. Her doctor then prescribed more potent pain relievers, including steroids and narcotics.

While pain medications are critical tools in treating pain and injury, many studies have demonstrated that in addition to addressing the multidimensional nature of chronic pain, treatment of the injured structure is critical to breaking the cycle leading to chronic pain and also associated mood problems caused by the pain.

Steroidal Anti-inflammatory Drugs

Steroids (corticosteroids or glucocorticoids) are synthetic forms of cor-tisol, which is produced naturally by the adrenal system in the body. One of the many roles corticosteroids play in the body is to regulate inflammation. Remember that NSAIDs work by inhibiting the enzymes COX-1 and COX-2, which promote the production of prostaglandins in the inflammatory response. Steroids decrease pain by interrupt-ing the inflammatory response much earlier in the chemical process than NSAIDs. They not only inhibit prostaglandin synthesis, they also inhibit the production of leukotrienes, another critical component of the inflammatory response. Leukotrienes play a role in the healing process by acting as transporters of the necessary cells (lymphocytes, which are specialized white blood cells) to the injured tissues and by controlling whether the blood vessels allow those cells to pass through the vessel walls and come in contact with the injured tissues. Lymphocytes are the body's defense system against infection, so they are critical when an injury involves an open wound. By controlling these two elements of the inflammatory response, steroids dramatically reduce inflammation and therefore reduce or eliminate pain.

When steroids are taken orally, they are called systemic. Systemic steroids are usually used in the short term (less than one month) and in moderate doses. Because of all the systems that corticosteroids affect in the body, when they are used longer than three months, a whole host of side effects can occur including:

- Increased appetite and weight gain
- Fatty deposits on the chest, face, upper back, and stomach
- Water and salt retention leading to swelling
- High blood pressure
- Diabetes
- Slowed wound healing
- Osteoporosis (thinning of the bones)
- Cataracts
- Acne
- Muscle weakness
- Thinning of the skin
- Increased susceptibility to infection
- Stomach ulcers
- Mood swings
- Psychological problems, including depression
- Adrenal suppression

If you are taking corticosteroids and need to stop taking them, your doctor will gradually reduce the dosage to permit your adrenal glands to reestablish natural production of cortisol. Stopping steroidal anti-inflammatory drugs too quickly can cause an adrenal crisis, so the dosage must taper off gradually. Doctors usually prescribe the lowest dose possible, but high-dose therapy (approximately 60 milligrams a day) is sometimes prescribed in severe cases of inflammatory disease such as rheumatoid arthritis and other related autoimmune diseases.

Commonly used steroids include betamethasone, cortisone, dexamethasone, methylprednisolone, prednisone, prednisolone, and triamcinolone.

Steroid Injections

Often when the RICE (rest, ice, compression, elevation) protocol, analgesics, or other medications fail to provide relief for a painful joint, steroid injections into or near the joint, at the very site of inflammation, are suggested. Please note that steroid injections and prolotherapy are *not* the same thing. In fact, they are effectual opposites: Steroid injections reduce inflammation of tendons, ligaments, and bursas; prolotherapy works by inducing inflammation to promote healing.

Steroid injections are particularly effective in treating conditions that involve chronic moderate to severe inflammation, such as bursitis or osteoarthritis. These types of injections are useful when the condition being controlled is chronic inflammation that is causing damage to the joint (as with osteoarthritis), but on

> Steroid injections reduce inflammation of tendons, ligaments, and bursas; prolotherapy works by inducing inflammation to promote healing.

the other hand, they can be harmful when used to treat an injury to soft tissues that need time and inflammation to heal fully and correctly. Small amounts of steroids injected into a joint can be useful, but the larger amounts commonly used cause all natural tissue repair to stop. And corticosteroids can further damage injured ligaments and tendons when they are injected repeatedly into a joint.

Cortisone injections are often used to treat bursitis. If you remember from chapter 1, bursas are fluid-filled sacs that are strategically placed around joints between tendons and bones to prevent trauma to the tendon. Imagine a rope constantly rubbing against a rough surface. How long do you think it will be before the rope becomes frayed and weak? The rope would last much longer sliding along an oiled and smooth surface. That is the purpose of the bursa — to prevent friction and the wear and tear that comes from it. Strategic injections of cortisone can quickly resolve bursitis, sometimes after only one or two treatments.

Corticosteroids, particularly when combined with an anesthetic (numbing agent), are often used in diagnostic injections. These injections can help doctors locate the exact source of the pain — the pain generator — especially among the many joints and discs of the spine. When a corticosteroid is injected into a joint (intra-articular injection) and the pain is substantially, albeit temporarily, improved, this is a good indication that the source of the pain is intra-articular (the soft tissues that exist within the joint) rather than extra-articular (the soft tissues around or outside the joint). This is a good use of steroid injections because the necessary dose is quite small.

If cortisone injections resolve the pain and swelling, then the tendon, ligament, or bursa was probably chronically inflamed. If the pain improves but does not resolve, then a tear may also have occurred. In this case, other treatment options should be considered to ensure proper healing. If an injection of cortisone and lidocaine (a local anesthetic) provides excellent, but temporary relief, then the pain is likely due solely to a soft tissue tear at the site, and prolotherapy would resolve the pain by promoting actual healing of the tear.

An open mind to the healing approach of injuries can prevent untold grief and expense. This is true for the treatment of lateral epicondylitis (also known as golfer's elbow) or medial epicondylitis (also known as tennis elbow), two commonly occurring repetitive use injuries we discussed in chapter 1. For these types of tendon injuries, a small steroid injection to the tendon often proves sufficient, particularly if the pain results solely from an inflammation of the tendon; however, if there is a partial tear, the pain will most likely come back. Any stress placed on the partially torn tendon will result in pain. Repeated steroid injections provide only temporary relief; meanwhile, this process also weakens the tendon and increases the likelihood of further tearing. At this point, the application of prolotherapy to the injured tendon can be very beneficial.

Usually, no more than three cortisone injections per year are injected into a weight-bearing joint because cortisone is known to weaken ligaments and tendons. In the past, athletes welcomed the temporary relief cortisone provided and sought repeated injections to allow them to continue playing. The result was weakened ligaments and tendons, which led to serious ruptures of the tendons that required surgical reattachment. Many promising athletic careers have ended after surgical intervention.

In addition to injecting steroids into joints, doctors may also use epidural steroid injections when treating back pain, particularly low back pain. Symptoms of some back conditions, such as spinal stenosis, can be greatly improved in many patients through the use of epidural injections because they reduce the inflammatory component. The period of pain relief from an epidural injection ranges from four to ten months. It is a simple outpatient procedure that may eliminate the need for major surgery and provide a safe and effective option for older patients who are not candidates for surgery.

While steroid injections are effective in treating some conditions, after a partial tear to a tendon or ligament, prolotherapy is the best option for full and correct healing. Your doctor might tell you that localizing an injection spares the rest of the body; however, frequent injections into the same joint can damage the cartilage and weaken bones, tendons, and ligaments. You then are left with more seriously weakened support structures, increased pain, little relief, and the promise of continued painful steroid injections. For chronic pain associated with weak ligaments and tendons, steroid injections only exacerbate the problem.

Nerve Blocks

Image-guided procedures allow precise delivery of medications to the pain generator. The goals of such treatments are to decrease inflammation and to accelerate tissue repair (healing), with the overall objective of providing powerful pain management. Another useful pain management tool is selective nerve blocks, which targets particular nerves carrying the pain signals from various diseased structures.

Nerve blocks involve injecting an anesthetic onto or near nerves to interrupt the message of pain between designated areas of the brain and your body. They literally block the pain message from reaching your brain and registering that an area of your body is hurt. Dentists, for example, often use nerve blocks for extensive dental work. As described in the section on corticosteroids, blocks are also sometimes used to provide diagnostic information and can help your doctor identify the source of your pain. For therapeutic purposes, nerve blocks should be used with caution and only in cases of severe pain because complications can occur. Sciatic nerve blocks, for example, have resulted in local anesthetic toxicity from the injection and permanent nerve injury.

Use of Other Medications to Treat Pain

You should always check with your doctor before taking drugs for pain relief, especially if a combination of prescription drugs is involved. Certain medicines, even those sold over the counter, may be unsafe during pregnancy, may conflict with other medications, may cause side effects including drowsiness, or may lead to

> You should always check with your doctor before taking drugs for pain relief, especially if a combination of prescription drugs is involved.

liver damage. Your doctor may select medications depending on the cause of your pain and the presence of other associated medical conditions, such as hypertension, diabetes, sleep apnea, or depression. These are usually prescribed based on whether the pain is inflammatory or neuropathic and are used in combination with several therapies tailored to fit the problem causing the pain.

The drugs most frequently used for pain relief include

- *Anticonvulsants*: Certain drugs primarily used to treat seizures may be employed in treating some types of nerve-generated pain and may also be prescribed with analgesics. They are also used to stabilize mood.

- *Antidepressants*: Some antidepressants — particularly tricyclic antidepressants such as amitriptyline, desipramine, or duloxetine — have been shown to relieve pain (independent of their effect on depression) and to assist with sleep. Antidepressants alter levels of brain chemicals to elevate mood and dull pain signals.

- *Opioids*: Drugs such as codeine, oxycodone, hydrocodone, and morphine are occasionally prescribed to manage severe acute and chronic back pain. Such medications should be used only for short periods of time and always under a physician's supervision. Side effects can include drowsiness, decreased reaction time, impaired judgment, and potential for addiction. Most respected authorities on pain management are convinced that chronic use of these drugs is detrimental to patients who suffer from back pain, adding to the possibility of their experiencing depression and even increasing their pain over time.

In very extreme cases of chronic pain, when no other treatment options have been effective, a doctor may use an implanted device that injects small doses at regular intervals into a person's system. Again, these are typically used only when all other treatment options (including surgery) have failed.

While pain medications can offer great relief, that relief is generally only temporary. Gary can testify to that. A World War II veteran, Gary suffered a back injury on the battlefield and later developed chronic back pain that persisted for many years. He saw many physicians for his pain, but none of the medications prescribed for him over the years were effective for very long. Over time, Gary became depressed and irritable. His mood changes interfered with his marriage and his relationships with friends and relatives. Despite his taking more powerful antidepressants and pain killers, his pain and mood changes did not improve, and he was now frustrated by the side effects of his medications, which he needed to take more frequently and in higher amounts to partially control his symptoms. Gary's story is far too common.

Natural Substances That Treat Inflammation and Pain

A number of natural products are marketed as beneficial in treating certain joint conditions, including osteoarthritis. They are meant to reduce swelling and pain as well as to increase physical functioning, such as flexibility and strength.

Glucosamine and chondroitin sulfate are recommended supplements for people with joint problems because they support the rebuilding of cartilage. Glucosamine is thought to prevent the destruction of joint cartilage due to the normal aging process and repetitive trauma. It may also contribute to the formation of new cartilage. Chondroitin is the most common proteoglycan that makes up cartilage. It makes sense that if we want to stimulate the body to make more cartilage we need to give the body the components necessary to produce it.

Methylsulfonylmethane (MSM) is a dietary supplement that has been shown in a double blind clinical trial to improve the pain, stiffness, physical function, and overall joint symptoms of individuals over the age of 40 diagnosed with knee osteoarthritis (Kim 2006). Although the exact mechanism by which MSM works is unknown, it is abundant in sulfur, an important component of the body's connective tissue. The joint pain may be improved, scientists believe, because of the beneficial sulfur MSM provides.

Dr. Barry Sears, in his book *The Anti-Inflammation Zone* (Regan, 2005) describes the benefits of using high doses of omega-3 fatty acids to treat chronic inflammation. Our typical American diet, according to Dr. Sears, can result in many chronic diseases that are related to inflammation, including diseases that cause joint pain. The problem primarily lies with the consumption of omega-6 fatty acids from animal fat and consumption of carbohydrates with high glycemic index ratings.

The hormones in our body that promote inflammation, such as prostaglandins and leukotrienes, are derived from arachidonic acid, which is an omega-6 fatty acid. Consumption of high levels of omega-6 can lead to an increase in arachidonic acid. In addition, high glycemic index carbohydrates increase insulin levels, and excess insulin results in an increase in arachidonic acid, further exacerbating the inflammation process in the body.

To combat chronic, unhealthy inflammation, Dr. Sears recommends high doses of omega-3 rich oils, particularly EPA from super-refined fish oils, which reduces the production of arachidonic acid and improves chronic joint pain. I recommend that all of my patients reduce their intake of omega-6s from animal fats, balance their consumption of carbohydrates, and take omega-3 supplements. To learn more about a low glycemic index diet, go to www.glycemicindex.com.

Some medications and dietary supplements include acids from the *Boswellia* genus of trees, which have shown promise in treating inflammation, particularly with osteoarthritis. It seems to inhibit the synthesis of leukotrienes, which are part of the inflammatory response. In addition, bromelain, an enzyme that occurs in pineapple, seems to help reduce inflammation, swelling, and pain. Though effective, bromelain may be accompanied by a variety of side effects, including vomiting, diarrhea, and possible allergic reactions.

Many natural substances have not been extensively tested to date, so their true efficacy is not known. Before trying a natural substance, consult with your doctor to make sure there aren't any potential side effects you should be aware of or any contraindications with medicines you are already taking.

Electrotherapy

Electrotherapy has been in use for more than a hundred years. Originally considered quack medicine, it is now touted for its ability to reduce both acute and chronic pain. Just before World War II, the U.S. War Department investigated the use of electrical stimulation to prevent and slow down muscle atrophy and to restore muscle mass and strength. The military eventually employed a form of therapy that allowed the passage of amperes through the muscle. It was determined that this form of exercise actually did facilitate recovery.

Today, several forms of electrotherapy are in use. For the types of problems we're discussing in this book, electrotherapy is typically employed by physical therapists. The most common system used to reduce pain is the transcutaneous electrical nerve stimulation (TENS) unit. It is effective in treating pain because the electrical signals it generates activate the opioid receptors in the central nervous system. A newer version of the TENS system is the percutaneous electrical nerve stimulation (PENS) system, which delivers electrical charges through tiny needles that are inserted over a painful area such as the lower back. In extreme cases of chronic pain, a nerve stimulation device may be implanted near the spine to repeatedly and consistently send electrical signals that activate the opioid receptors.

Another important system uses either electro muscle stimulation (EMS) or neuro-muscular electro stimulation (NMES) to trigger muscle contraction through electric stimulation. Medical professionals recommend this system mainly to calm muscle spasms, rehabilitate and reeducate muscles that have become atrophied, increase or restore range of motion, and facilitate recovery from surgery or medical therapy.

EMS or NMES involves applying an adhesive electrode to the skin through which electrical stimulation is then transmitted to nerves and muscles. This stimulation is generally painless. In particular, EMS causes the muscles to contract and release, which adds strength and functionality to injured soft tissue. Side effects from this form of stimulation are rare; however, minor allergic reactions from the adhesive pads have occurred. This type of electrical stimulation should not be used over the heart, the uterus in pregnant women, or infections or malignancies.

While EMS and NMES have proven to be beneficial in treating pain and in resolving muscular problems, they don't necessarily help resolve other soft tissue injuries. Sometimes, when there is an injury to a tendon or a ligament, the surrounding muscles become stiff or spasm. The chronic muscle spasm can in turn pull on the injured tendon, resulting in increased pain. Healing the injured tendon contributes to the resolution of the muscle spasm, as well.

Nerve Destruction

As described in chapter 2, some pain is primarily generated by nerve damage. And some pain is exacerbated or caused by nerves misfiring after trauma, sending pain signals when no pain generator exists. In these cases, localized nerve destruction can eliminate the pain. In the past, nerves were severed surgically. For the most part, this approach has been abandoned because it was sometimes associated with abnormal and painful regrowth of the nerve fibers. The abnormal regrowth, called neuroma, sometimes led to a paradoxical *increase* in pain severity.

To reduce this and other potential complications, radiofrequency ablation was developed to treat sensory nerves more accurately and effectively. Radiofrequency current, when delivered to tissues, is converted to heat, which is highly controlled in space and intensity. Radiofrequency is thus used to treat a small volume of nerve tissue, thereby disrupting transmission of pain signals along a specific nerve. With the help of imaging techniques, the procedure can reduce pain in targeted areas, leaving other nerves and the supporting structures of the treated nerve intact and preventing neuroma formation. Radiofrequency therapy has become a mainstream approach in pain medicine, providing a safe, proven means of treating chronic pain.

When used in the facet joints of the spine, this process is called facet denervation. First, the physician identifies the facet joint that is causing the pain by numbing the nerves carrying the pain signals from specific facets. Once the culprit joint or joints are identified, these nerves can be treated using radiofrequency lesioning. When the technique is expertly performed, it causes little discomfort; it is safe and should not damage important nerves such as those carrying motor commands to the muscles.

Remember the World War II veteran Gary? He was eventually diagnosed with painful facet arthropathy (a form of arthritis affecting the facet joints of the spine). Gary underwent a treatment in which the medial branch nerves of the spine (the nerves that carry the sensations and pain signals from the facets) were stunned using radiofrequency. Although it took four treatments to achieve pain control, Gary's pain began to decrease after a few weeks of therapy, and his negative mood dramatically improved. His relationships were revitalized; according to his wife, he was a different person altogether. He could also reduce the number and dosages of medications needed to control his pain.

Another form of nerve destruction used in the discs of the spine is intradiscal electrothermoplasty. In this procedure, a wire is temporarily inserted into a disc. The wire is then heated, destroying the sensory nerves. This procedure cannot be used on severely degenerated discs.

While nerve destruction can be an effective treatment for extreme pain, permanently destroying nerves can result in other nerves picking up the sensory message. Not only can the pain return, but complications can result from the procedure as well.

Many options are available for you to consider when you are in pain. The treatments outlined in this chapter are used to treat both acute pain and chronic pain during the healing process. Regardless of the pain treatment options you have tried or are considering, you must treat the underlying problem if you want to achieve permanent healing and lasting pain relief.

Chapter 6

Noninvasive Options for Treating the Injury

Michele was a young woman who had previously undergone back surgery for scoliosis, during which a surgeon inserted metal rods to help her spine hold a straight alignment. Her back surgery had been very successful, and she had returned to an active lifestyle shortly thereafter. Over the years, however, Michele began to experience increasing pain in her left buttock. She had to give up one of her favorite pastimes, bowling, because it had become too painful to play. Even simple walking had become limited: She could not walk for longer than thirty minutes. Pain radiated down her leg as a result of compression of the sciatic nerve as it passed through the piriformis muscle (a gluteal muscle that runs from the sacrum outward through the SI joint). No medication was effective at relieving her chronic pain, and Michele was reduced to lying down when the pain became intolerable.

Although her back surgery for scoliosis had been necessary and successful, it nonetheless resulted in increased stress on her left SI joint and thus her piriformis muscle. Repeated visits to neurosurgeons resulted in no treatments that relieved her pain. No one wanted to touch the Harrington rods placed in her back many years earlier. Although the rods prevented further deterioration of her spine from the scoliosis and improved that condition itself, they did not make her back "normal."

Because so many options for healing a joint or back injury are available today, doctors must consult with their patients to determine which solution will work best at each stage of the treatment process. But every doctor's experiences are different. Some physicians believe that physical therapy is the cure for almost every injury. Others have faith in chiropractic intervention. Still others consider it prudent to immediately refer their patients to orthopedic specialists or surgeons.

> Every doctor should be searching for ways to treat the underlying problem—the pain generator—and not just to manage the pain.

Therefore, *you* must take the initiative and examine all of the available treatments in order to make a choice that's right for *you*. Obviously, the less invasive the treatment, the better your chances are for immediate as well as long-term recovery. Primary care physicians have a duty to consider all of the less-invasive options before progressing to more-invasive options. And every doctor should be searching for ways to treat the underlying problem—the pain generator—and not just to manage the pain.

To support this process, I developed an algorithm (that is, a procedure or method used to solve a problem) that helps me determine the most appropriate course of treatment for each patient I see with a joint or back soft tissue injury. My algorithm is shown in figure 6.1.

Most types of injuries or medical problems have treatment algorithms that are put forth by medical associations, published in journals, or produced by the government health agencies. These algorithms are

Figure 6.1: Treatment Algorithm for Joint and Back Injuries

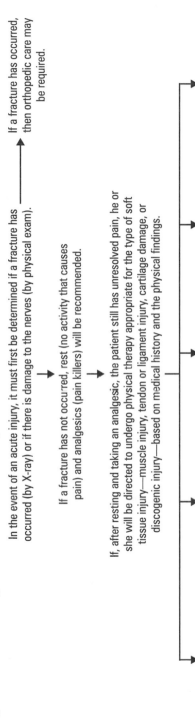

In the event of an acute injury, it must first be determined if a fracture has occurred (by X-ray) or if there is damage to the nerves (by physical exam).

If a fracture has occurred, then orthopedic care may be required.

If a fracture has not occurred, rest (no activity that causes pain) and analgesics (pain killers) will be recommended.

If, after resting and taking an analgesic, the patient still has unresolved pain, he or she will be directed to undergo physical therapy appropriate for the type of soft tissue injury—muscle injury, tendon or ligament injury, cartilage damage, or discogenic injury—based on medical history and the physical findings.

If a muscle injury is diagnosed, the patient will be treated with one or more of the following: massage/myofascial release, trigger point injections, strain/counterstrain technique, or botulinum toxin.

If there is ligament damage, treatment will be based on the extent of damage. If the damage is minimal, the patient can be treated with rest, bracing, and physical therapy. If the damage is more extensive, prolotherapy/regenerative injection techniques will be recommended.

If there is tendon damage and subsequent sprain, prolotherapy will be provided, with other regenerative injection therapies, such as platelet-rich plasma injections, as an option.

If there is cartilage damage, the patient will be provided prolotherapy with hyaluronic acid (synvisc).

If there is both ligament and tendon damage with discogenic injury (injury to the discs of the spine), chiropractic manipulation will be recommended.

If the problem is unresolved through chiropractic manipulation or prolotherapy, evaluation by an interventional pain specialist will be considered.

If there is spinal nerve compression or the problem is unresolved, surgical evaluation will be recommended.

generally based on past research and the experience of a committee of experts in the field. Insurance companies will often refer to them to help them determine if a requested test or treatment is reasonable or recommended for a given condition. The problem is that so few physicians are well trained in diagnosing and treating soft tissue injuries, soft tissue injuries are hard to clearly identify through testing, and most standard algorithms don't take all available options for treatment into account. This is why I have developed my algorithm. It incorporates the best medical recommendations from the usual standards of care but goes a step further to incorporate tests and treatments that should be considered before more drastic treatment measures are taken. While it can take years to update standard algorithms in the medical community, I keep mine up to date with the latest medical research.

Let's take a look at some of the noninvasive treatments that can support the healing process.

Physical Therapy

The goal of physical therapy — a rehabilitation treatment — is to maintain and restore maximum physical functioning of the body. Physical therapists work with clients who have been injured, who have physical diseases, or whose functional ability is limited in some other way. In many instances, physical therapy can promote healing after an injury and can also reduce or resolve pain.

Most people who are treated by a physical therapist have been referred to this type of specialist by their primary care physician. This is usually done after a course of the RICE protocol and pain medications or anti-inflammatory drugs fail to resolve an injury. Physicians recommend physical therapy when it is clear that a person's functional abilities are suffering because of the injury.

A physical therapist's primary tool is controlled and directed physical exercises that are designed to increase the range of motion and strengthen weakened areas. As mentioned briefly in chapter 1, therapists also sometimes use such other treatments as ice and heat, electrical stimulation of muscles, massage, and ultrasound. During a typical course of physical therapy, a patient performs exercises under the guidance of a therapist or assistant and is also given homework— exercises to do at home on a regular basis.

Physical therapists are licensed medical professionals who hold either a master's degree or a doctorate in physical therapy. Some specialize in specific areas of therapy including neurological, orthopedic, and pediatric.

When done properly, physical therapy is a low-risk treatment to aid the body in recuperating from a soft tissue injury. It is most effective early in the healing process, soon after an injury has been sustained. Some injuries are minor enough to need only time in order to heal, but other injuries should be treated with physical therapy immediately. Physical therapy is also very useful in keeping you moving and exercising after surgery to repair severely damaged tissues. In these cases, physical therapy is essential for full healing and recovery.

Physical therapy can occasionally be harmful, but only when the therapist involved does not practice good, safe protocols for diagnosis and treatment. If you are working with a therapist who takes the same approach to every injury, employing the same treatment, and doesn't take the time to fully and correctly diagnose the problem and identify the specific soft tissues involved, then the treatment is unlikely to be beneficial and may actually hinder the healing process.

The McKenzie Method

Another very important component in the treatment of joint pain is exercise. I'm not referring to just any exercise, but to exercises specifically designed for your particular problem. Robin McKenzie is a physical therapist who discovered the effectiveness of focused exercises designed to extend the spine in relieving low back and neck pain.

Much research has been performed to verify the usefulness of these exercises in both diagnosis and treatment.

The McKenzie Method requires the application of seven exercises for the neck and seven exercises for the back, as well as postural correction. Robin McKenzie believes that most low back and neck pain results from persistent overstretching of the ligaments and surrounding soft tissue, primarily attributed to poor posture. Of course trauma and repetitive overuse are also common causes of ligament sprain. McKenzie also attributes some disc problems to ligament laxity.

It is my belief that the McKenzie Method should be a treatment component of every back injury, particularly considering the fact that many back problems can be completely resolved with physical therapy methods.

Acupuncture

Acupuncture is one of the world's oldest healing practices. Part of traditional Chinese medicine, it is more widely accepted in Western medicine now than it has ever been and is sometimes prescribed when other methods of pain management and healing have failed. It is used primarily as a supplemental therapy for soft tissue injuries.

The full effects of acupuncture are not completely understood by the scientific community and the body of evidence to support the effectiveness of acupuncture, particularly in treating pain, is controversial. Yet many in the medical community believe that it is beneficial and recommend it to the people they treat for certain conditions, and in some hospitals it is being used to induce labor, treat pain, improve symptoms of chronic illness, and to treat many other conditions.

Acupuncture involves stimulating specific points on the body through a variety of techniques. It most often involves penetrating the skin with a thin metallic needle that is manipulated by either the hands or electrical stimulation. Most people feel minimal or no pain when the needles are inserted. The objective is to achieve a balance of *yin* and *yang*, two opposing forces: *Yin* representing the cold, slow, or passive principle; and *yang* representing the hot, excited, or active principle. Imbalances can lead to blockages in the flow of vital energy, or *qi* (sometimes spelled *chi*). Acupuncture unblocks *qi* at points in the body where the pathway for the flow of energy is blocked. There are approximately two thousand acupuncture points and fifteen to twenty meridians, or pathways, in the body.

Few complications or side effects result from acupuncture; however, inadequate sterilization of needles can result in infection, and improper delivery can puncture organs. Practitioners should use a new set of disposable needles for each patient. In addition, all injection sites should be swabbed with a disinfectant before the needles are inserted. It is therefore imperative to find a qualified practitioner. Most states require acupuncturists to be licensed, but requirements and oversight vary from state to state.

Before seeking relief for pain from an acupuncturist, be sure you have first had a diagnosis from a medical doctor. You may wish to ask your diagnosing physician whether acupuncture treatments could help your condition. Your physician may also be able to recommend an acupuncturist who has experience working with people with your condition.

Massage Therapy

Massage therapists are trained specifically to deal with musculoskel-etal and myofascial pain syndromes—that is, any pains involving the muscles and other soft tissues. They manipulate soft tissue and muscle to relieve pain in those areas. The primary focus is on relaxing tight or spasming muscles. This in turn relieves pressure on the surrounding connective tissue. Like other treatments described in this chapter, massage therapy may not resolve a soft tissue injury, but it can nevertheless be a beneficial part of the treatment process.

Massage therapy can be highly effective in relieving pain and tension resulting from whiplash injuries. Symptoms of whiplash include having a stiff neck, muscle pain, headaches, dizziness, and shoulder and back pain. Massage helps relax the muscles and restores balance to the musculoskeletal system. Furthermore, massage can restore and enhance range of motion, increase circulation, and prevent and break down the formation of scar tissue.

Strain/Counterstrain Technique

Strain/counterstrain is not a treatment for injured or damaged soft tissues. Rather, it is a treatment intended to resolve aberrant neuromuscular reflexes and positioning that are causing muscle spasms. In other words, the nerves in the muscle are misfiring and sending signals to the brain to keep the muscle contracted when it should not be.

Strain/counterstrain techniques are considered passive positional therapy: One element of the therapy is to position the body in such a way as to help the muscles relax. When a massage therapist is able to identify the correct positioning and allow the muscles to relax, the muscles will begin to reset to their natural positions. In a contribution to the book *Rational Manual Therapies* (1992), Randall S. Kusunose, an expert on strain/counterstrain techniques, described the biological process as follows:

> What strain and counterstrain attempts to accomplish with its position of comfort is to relax the muscle spasm by reducing aberrant afferent [neuron] flow from the muscle spindle. This is accomplished by mimicking the original strain position or applying a "counterstrain." By passively mimicking the original strain position, the operator moves the joint in a direction of ease and . . . shortens the involved muscle. Holding for 90 seconds allows the spindle to slow down its afferent [neuron] firing frequency. Returning to neutral in a

slow and deliberate manner avoids reexciting the previously spasmed muscles. (331)

Once the natural position is achieved, the massage therapist then begins to stretch and manipulate the muscle to resolve any remaining tense fibers (or trigger points), helping the patient achieve lasting correct muscle positioning and function. The massage of the muscle fibers is directed by the location of myofascial trigger points—small zones of tense, tender muscle and fascial tissue.

Strain/counterstrain is often used when a person has a musculoskeletal imbalance, such as a high hip or high shoulder. Resolving improper muscle contraction and incorrect positioning can be very helpful in these situations, allowing the patient to achieve balance and, therefore, pain relief.

Myofascial Release

Myofascial release is a soft tissue therapy that is similar to massage, although the goals and techniques are different. The fascia of the body is the web of interconnected tissues that support the body's structure. The deep fascia includes tendons, ligaments, joint capsules, and other connective tissues. The goal of myofascial release is to loosen the fibers of the various fascia components by stretching them and breaking bonds that have formed between connective tissues and other soft tissues through scarring, improper healing of injuries, or repeatedly misusing those body tissues (as can result from poor posture, excessive time spent working at a computer, etc.).

Some people refer to this work as deep tissue massage therapy, but the two practices are different because myofascial release focuses on tendons, ligaments, and other structures that are tight, are mispositioned, or have bonded with other structures in a way that impedes their full function. Myofascial release can be quite painful at the time that it is being done, but the effects tend to be long lasting and, for some people, offer immediate relief for certain conditions.

Botulinum Toxin

Let's return to Michele's story. Although a pain in the hips or buttocks may result from weakened ligaments of the SI joint, for Michele the pain was also tied to the piriformis muscle. Trigger point injections with lidocaine were very effective at relieving her pain, but that relief would last just ten to fourteen days. Because Michele's condition wasn't improving and she was only achieving temporary relief, I began injecting botulinum toxin into the muscle. Botulinum toxin, popularly known as Botox, is one of the newest methods being used to treat stubborn cases of muscle spasm. Although initially used on muscles to correct crossed eyes and eyelid tics, its safety record permitted its use for many other conditions, among them relaxing muscles on the forehead and around the eyes, making wrinkles disappear. Myobloc is the trade name of another type of botulinum toxin approved for use in cases of cervical dystonia (severe muscle spasms in the neck), but may also be used to treat conditions like Michele's, where muscle spasms are the root cause of the pain.

Myobloc can be used for patients who continue to experience chronic aches and tightness in their muscles. Injecting lidocaine into the trigger points or taut muscle cords may be effective and may be much less expensive than Myobloc. But, as was the case with Michele, when lidocaine trigger point injections prove effective but too short lasting, Myobloc can be given to prolong the relief, possibly even permanently.

More research is being done to determine what conditions are best treated with Myobloc, but in my experience, it has proven to be most effective in treating an under-recognized condition known as piriformis muscle syndrome, or severe spasm of the piriformis muscle. This relatively rare diagnosis occurs most often in cyclists and skaters who overuse this muscle, as well as from trauma. While the piriformis muscle syndrome may be accompanied by an SI joint dysfunction, the muscle spasm may persist even if the joint dysfunction is resolved. By squeezing the sciatic nerve, which passes through this muscle, this severe spasm can result in pain. The pain is distributed along the sciatic nerve to the back of the buttock and thigh. This occurs most often in patients who have already undergone back surgery, possibly from the increased stress placed on the muscle and the increased instability resulting from the surgery.

Piriformis muscle syndrome may be diagnosed by confirming the presence of a tender sausage-like mass over the muscle. Movements that stretch the piriformis muscle may also illicit pain. Injecting the piriformis muscle with an anesthetic can confirm a diagnosis and determine the route of treatment. Frequently, however, the pain recurs because the muscle spasm is not permanently relieved. Surgical release (cutting the muscle) used to be the only option in recalcitrant cases, but now Myobloc can be used. It paralyzes the muscle fibers and forces the muscle to relax. Myobloc injections may effect a permanent cure, but the muscle spasms often return in three to four months, necessitating repetitive treatments.

Another condition that can be treated with Myobloc is dystonia. Dystonia is a movement disorder that causes involuntary muscle contractions. In the case of idiopathic cervical (neck) dystonia, it is believed that a defect in the brain stem causes severe spasm of various cervical muscles. This chronic contracture can cause severe pain and make it impossible to turn or move the neck normally. Injections of Myobloc into the affected muscles provides relief within a few days and lasts three to four months before reapplication is necessary.

Within days of the first Myobloc treatment, Michele felt even more complete pain relief than with the lidocaine, and the effects lasted much longer. She was able to resume normal activities, including walking and standing for long periods of time throughout the day. After a few weeks of increased activities, Michele began to experience left low back pain. Because of the connection between the piriformis muscle and the

SI joint, it wasn't surprising that an examination revealed left SI joint laxity. We started a prolotherapy regimen, and she felt complete relief with just two treatments. Strengthening her SI joint may improve the piriformis muscle spasms or resolve them entirely.

Chiropractic Therapy

Chiropractic therapy has been practiced for more than one hundred years. It is one of the safest, noninvasive treatments available for back, neck, and limb pain, as well as other neuromusculoskeletal problems.

Chiropractors are licensed medical professionals. They can diagnose and treat musculoskeletal and nervous system disorders, but they cannot prescribe medications or perform surgery. If they cannot treat an injury or condition, chiropractors usually refer patients to a medical specialist.

Misalignment of a vertebra (known as a subluxation) can place pressure on spinal nerves, causing pain. By adjusting the spine, the chiropractor can return the vertebra to the proper position in the spinal column. In addition, chiropractic work can help alleviate pain or stiffness in the back, neck, shoulders, arms, hands, hips, legs, knees, and feet. It is also useful for some types of migraine headaches, mild forms of scoliosis, sciatica, whiplash, sports injuries, arthritis, bursitis, tendinitis, and fibromyalgia. During the hands-on therapeutic adjustment, pockets of gas are released from the joints, accounting for the popping sound that sometimes occurs.

If you have been suffering from an injury for some time, you probably favor the part of your body that is injured. When you do this, you create misalignment in your body. Regardless of what other types of treatment you use to treat the injury, you may want to consider chiropractic therapy to help your body return to normal alignment and functioning.

Chiropractors, like many other medical professionals, maintain that the body has self-healing properties and that structural irregularity and impeded function can affect overall health. The therapy aims to restore function and health by normalizing the skeletal and muscular structure. By returning your body to its normal shape and working order, chiropractors believe when the pain is removed, your health improves.

In addition to spinal manipulation, chiropractors may use other treatments such as ice and heat, electrical stimulation, rehabilitative exercises, and dietary and vitamin supplements. Any time a dietary supplement is recommended or provided, be sure to let your physician know because supplements can interact with drugs you may already be taking.

Chiropractic therapy is relatively risk free, but it can cause headaches, temporary fatigue, and muscle aches in treated areas. Soreness or achiness usually fades within twenty-four hours. When used with prolotherapy, chiropractic therapy can help restore movement while maintaining spinal alignment. If chiropractic adjustments provide only temporary relief, there may be an underlying problem of ligament laxity that is allowing your spine to slip out of alignment. If that is the case, regenerative injection therapies, such as prolotherapy, can result in permanent relief.

Remember Nancy from the previous chapter, the woman who was involved in three major car accidents? She went to a chiropractor for an extended period of time. For a while, his treatments helped. But on one visit to his office, the adjustment caused Nancy more pain. She realized that although it was helpful, the chiropractic adjustment did not actually solve her underlying problems.

Then Nancy learned about prolotherapy. She made her first appointment in June 2003. It was her last hope, and she told the doctor so. From the very first injection in Nancy's neck, her range of motion increased. For several months, Nancy received prolotherapy, and her improvements were continuous. That year, she actually enjoyed making dinner for both Thanksgiving and Christmas and entertaining company. In February 2004, Nancy visited Disney World again, walked all day, and then drove home. Because her condition was so severe, and because such a long time had elapsed between the injuries and the prolotherapy, she required an extensive course of treatment. (This is unusual as you'll see when I discuss the average course of treatment in chapters 7 and 8.) Ultimately, prolotherapy changed Nancy's life.

Spinal Decompression Therapy

Spinal decompression therapy is a relatively new form of treatment that uses traction to gently stretch the spine and relieve pressure on the discs. It is used to treat disc injuries and is typically performed by chiropractors. When the spine is stretched, not only is the pressure on the discs relieved, but a vacuum or negative pressure is also created within the disc (negative intradiscal pressure). This negative pressure causes the center of the disc that may be bulging outward to retract and relieves pressure on the nerves of the spine. And like movement in a joint that promotes the distribution of necessary nutrients and elements of healing and repair, the negative pressure helps diffuse oxygen and nutrient-rich fluids from the outer cells of the disc to the inner cells, promoting repair, healing, and strengthening.

The machine that creates the decompression has a table that you lie on (either on your back or your stomach). Straps around the waist and chest or rubber supports behind the neck hold you in place while the table does the work of stretching the spine and then relaxing it, over and over again in a pulsating rhythm. Typically the treatment causes no pain. One problem with this approach is that high-quality evidence of efficacy is missing. The changes with each decompression are microscopic, but over four to six weeks of treatment, the cumulative effects can be dramatic in occasional patients.

Some people are not good candidates for this treatment. If you have a spinal tumor, vertebral fractures, metal implants, rods, or screws in your spine, advanced osteoporosis, or are pregnant, you cannot use this therapy.

When you are in pain or are suffering from an injury, there are many treatment options. Some treatments work well when used in tandem with other treatments, and some practitioners use a combination of methods to ensure that all aspects of a physical problem are being addressed. In the next chapter, I explain the more advanced treatments of regenerative injection therapies.

Chapter 7

Regenerative Injection Therapies

Gino was a student of judo for a number of years, and he became quite accomplished in that sport. In college, he was invited to join the judo team, and later on Gino decided to join the professional circuit as well. But he had been having problems with his ankles, particularly his right one. His ankle was weak, and none of the therapies he tried—medications, support straps, physical therapy—seemed to be adequate in keeping it stable. After each series of matches, his right ankle would be swollen and painful. His doctors told him that his ligaments were not strong enough to keep his ankle joint stable and they recommended surgery. But Gino didn't want to undergo surgery, so he quit competing. Over time, the condition got worse. After experiencing ten years of pain and numerous twisted ankles, he stopped participating in all sports. They were simply no longer pleasurable activities.

During a trip to Argentina to visit his family, Gino was driving cattle on horseback on their ranch. The horse spooked and Gino tried to control him, but they both went down; the horse landed on Gino's right leg. There was a pop in his ankle, followed by immediate numbness and swelling. Gino thought that this time, he wouldn't be able to avoid surgery.

When, like Gino, you've spent money on physical therapy or massage therapy and you've seen little improvement of a weakened joint or a low back pain, you feel emotionally and financially frustrated. If a doctor you trust then tells you that the only option is surgery if you want lasting relief and an active life, you expect that you're probably in for more pain, a long recovery time, and a lot more money. Do you have any other options?

In chapter 6, I described a number of preliminary or noninvasive therapies that are frequently recommended by physicians to treat muscle, tendon, ligament, and disc injuries. But for many people, these therapies provide only temporary relief because an underlying soft tissue problem, often involving the tendons or ligaments, is not being resolved. In this chapter, I discuss various types of regenerative injection therapies—that is, therapies that involve injections into soft tissues to promote the healing, growth, and strengthening of those structures.

Dry Needling

Dry needling is a therapy that involves piercing soft tissue with a very thin solid needle (not an injection needle) to cause small injury to or bleeding in the soft tissue. Although this therapy does not involve injecting any substance into the body, it causes the regeneration of damaged or weakened tissues. Dry needling works because the localized bleeding delivers growth factors to the area of injury.

Dry needling a tendon or ligament is the most basic form of proliferative injection techniques (a very basic form of prolotherapy). It results in local inflammation and the delivery of platelets that contain growth factors to the area to promote healing and tissue repair. While some compare dry needling to acupuncture, the practices are different. Dry needling typically involves actually piercing the soft tissue structures that are injured rather than putting needles into meridian points. Dry needling is often performed by a physician or a physical therapist.

The December 1, 2008, issue of *U.S. News & World Report* contained an article by Alan Mozes titled "New Twist on Treatment of Foot Pain." In it Mozes reported on a presentation by Dr. Luca Sconfienza at the annual meeting of the Radiological Society of North America in which Sconfienza detailed the findings of a study on the use of a therapy that combined dry needling and steroid injections to treat plantar fasciitis, a painful condition caused by excessive wear to the plantar fascia, which connects your heel bone to your toes and supports the arch of your foot. The treatment was 95 percent effective in relieving heel pain. Neither treatment has been shown to be that effective when used by itself. The study doctors used ultrasound guidance to inject a small amount of steroids around, but not into, the plantar fascia because the steroids would seriously damage the fascia if injected directly into it. To ensure that the condition did not return, the doctors recommended physical therapy and the use of orthotics. In this study, interventional radiologists — that is, radiologists who administer treatments to resolve injuries rather than strictly perform diagnostic procedures — administered the treatment.

In treating muscle pain and spasm, dry needling may be called trigger point dry needling or intramuscular stimulation. The needle is used to pierce the muscle tissue at the myofascial trigger point, or knot, that is created by the shortening of the muscle after injury or trauma or with chronic spasm. The needle desensitizes the area by causing a small cramp. This allows the nerves to stop sending the message to the brain to contract the muscle, thereby causing the muscle to relax. Essentially, it stops a dysfunctional pattern of behavior in the muscle tissue. For some, this treatment provides an immediate sense of relief with little pain. For others, it may be more painful and may require multiple treatments. In this context, dry needling may be performed by acupuncturists or by physical therapists, depending on state regulations. Dry needling may also be combined with electrical stimulation (running an electrical charge through the needle to reach deep into the muscle) to achieve deep and stronger stimulation of the muscle fibers and peripheral nerves.

Myofascial trigger points may consist of multiple contraction knots. They can cause pain locally, particularly when stimulated with pressure, but they can also refer pain to more distant locations (recall the discussion of referred pain patterns from chapter 2). Myofascial trigger points can also cause muscle weakness, limited range of motion, and altered muscle activation patterns, in which the nerve signals that go back and forth to the brain are interrupted and cause incorrect muscle activity.

Prolotherapy

As described earlier in the book, prolotherapy involves a series of injections that produce an inflammatory response in injured tissues to promote the growth of normal cells and tissues, which results in healing the area more completely. Recall the description of the healing process in chapter 1: It all begins with inflammation. Unlike steroid injections, which suppress inflammation, or anesthetics, which treat pain by numbing the area, the substances used in the prolotherapy injections promote inflammation. Inflammation causes blood to rush to the site, stimulating the production and delivery of growth factors that promote healing to cartilage, tendons, and ligaments—all of which have poor blood supplies and cannot heal without the inflammatory boost. Because inflammation is essential to healing during prolotherapy, anti-inflammatory substances are not recommended during treatment. Table 3.1 lists commonly used anti-inflammatory drugs to be avoided during prolotherapy.

So, why is prolotherapy the best solution to heal an injury in many cases? First of all, prolotherapy actually promotes the healing process: It doesn't just mask the pain or the problem; it actually helps resolve them in many cases. Second, prolotherapy is one of the few solutions available to people with chronic pain. Although most patients with chronic joint and back pain are told that it will be a part of their lives forever, prolotherapy is proving over and over again that chronic pain is not a life sentence. Third, prolotherapy can improve a patient's range of motion. With joint injury, the patient's ability to move and use the joint is hindered, often to the point of disability. But prolotherapy directly strengthens the ligaments and tendons so that the injured person can have normal use of his or her joint or back. Finally, prolotherapy offers a cure for an underlying condition and in many cases, is less expensive than other regenerative injection therapies, and can help you avoid surgery. Fortunately, the list of injuries or conditions for which prolotherapy is an effective form of treatment is quite extensive. Refer to the Frequently Asked Questions About Prolotherapy section on the next page for a list of some of them.

The injections associated with prolotherapy are administered over the course of weeks or months. Your physician determines the time frame, the number of injections, and the frequency of office visits based on the severity of your condition, the length of time you have been debilitated or in pain, and your response to initial injections. How your body handles the injections, the change in your pain level, and the change in your abilities and range of motion influences the amount of prolotherapy you need. That said, the average prolotherapy course is six to eight treatments, and some people find relief after just two.

Some physicians inject one specific area at each visit. Others use a holistic approach and provide balanced injections to surrounding areas that may also be affected. A whiplash victim may receive injections to the cervical area alone or to the cervical area, back, and hip because all of these areas were affected by the injury: Muscles in several areas of the body tend to compensate in response to an injury in one area. A physician will

> The average prolotherapy course is six to eight treatments, and some people find relief after just two.

FREQUENTLY ASKED QUESTIONS

What is prolotherapy?

Prolotherapy is a treatment that uses a series of injections to produce inflammation in and around injured tissue. The injection components irritate cells and put into action what is called the inflammatory cascade. Inflammation is a natural response of the body—it stimulates the production and delivery of growth factors through the blood stream that promote healing of injured tissues. Ligaments and other soft tissues have poor blood supplies. Thus, healing in these areas is difficult and often incomplete. By inducing inflammation after the body's natural healing response has ceased, prolotherapy furthers the repair of tissues that may have healed poorly or incompletely. What were once lax and loose ligaments and tendons become taught and renewed, thus stabilizing joints that were hypermobile and eliminating stress on surrounding structures, such as muscles.

Is prolotherapy a proven, medical technique?

Many studies have been conducted highlighting the benefits of prolotherapy, and more are being conducted every day. It is used by some hospitals in the Mayo Clinic system. It has been in use for more than fifty years, and hundreds of physicians offer it to their patients across the country.

What conditions usually respond well to prolotherapy?

If you seek to lessen or eliminate chronic pain, improve your range of motion, and avoid surgery, prolotherapy might be your best option. Some specific injuries or conditions that can be treated successfully with prolotherapy include:

- Sprain of the ligaments in any joint
- Tendinosis or deterioration of the tendon fibers
- Joint instability due to ligament laxity, as a result of injury, repetitive stress or misuse, or an underlying medical condition, such as Ehlers-Danlos syndrome
- Medial or lateral epicondylitis (tennis elbow or golfer's elbow)
- Migraines or headaches associated with ligament injury or laxity in the cervical spine, such as whiplash
- Lower back pain associated with ligament injury or laxity in the lumbar spine
- Chronic spasming of the piriformis muscle (by treating the ligaments and tendons of the sacroiliac joint)
- Sacroiliac joint pain and instability
- Repetitive sprain or strain conditions
- Spinal pain
- Barre-Lieou syndrome
- Chronic dislocation

- Hyperextension or hyperflexion injuries
- Shoulder and neck pain (cervicobrachial syndrome resulting from weakened ligaments in the cervical spine and neck)
- Myofascial pain syndrome
- Whiplash injuries
- Facet joint pain
- Plantar fasciitis
- Some of the pain resulting from scoliosis
- Carpal tunnel syndrome
- Sciatica-like pain
- Rotator cuff injury
- Chronic subluxations of the vertebrae

Will prolotherapy work where other treatments have failed?
Prolotherapy may be the treatment of choice for patients who fail to improve after physical therapy, chiropractic or osteopathic manipulations, steroid injections, or surgical interventions for the conditions listed, or when any of these modalities are contraindicated (that is, not recommended) for a condition.

Will prolotherapy hurt?
No more than any injection. You might feel some stiffness where you were injected, and in some cases, your physician will tell you to take acetaminophen (such as Tylenol). But by no means should you take anti-inflammatory drugs (see chapter 3), because suppressing inflammation provides only temporary relief and slows or stops the healing response initiated by the prolotherapy injections.

How long will it take before I feel better?
Pain leaves only when all of the pain generators have been identified and treated. Soft tissue injuries—especially years after an initial injury—often masquerade as neurological problems. It sometimes takes time to get to the source of the problem to eliminate it. Some patients, however, might begin to feel a difference after the first treatment, and on average, most prolotherapy courses involve six to eight treatments. It all depends on the severity of your case and the amount of time you have been in pain.

Where can I find more information about prolotherapy?
You can find more information about prolotherapy online and in medical articles listed on PubMed.com, a service of the U.S. National Library of Medicine, and in publications such as *Practical Pain Management, Journal of Prolotherapy, Spine,* and others that deal with joint problems.

be able to decide where you need the most injections and what areas should be treated to provide the fastest relief.

When Gino came back to Texas after his trip to Argentina, he came to see me. He gave me his complete history and told me about his recent injury. I knew right away that prolotherapy could help him. Gino received four treatments in his right ankle and a year later came back for treatment of his left ankle. His ankles twist less often, are much less painful, and he's even able to play soccer again. He told me that he couldn't believe that after ten years of living with pain and seeing a dozen specialists, a family practitioner with a simple treatment resolved his problem.

I describe prolotherapy in depth in the next chapter.

Platelet-Rich Plasma Tissue Grafting

Note: This section was contributed by Edward Magaziner, MD, Board Certified in Physical Medicine and Rehabilitation, Pain Medicine, and Minimally Invasive Spine Surgery; Medical Director of the Center for Spine Sports Pain Management and Orthopedic Regenerative Medicine; Assistant Professor at New York Medical College; and Clinical Professor at Robert Wood Johnson University Medical School.

This technique involves injecting platelet-rich plasma (PRP) — also known as autologous platelet concentrate, platelet leukocyte gel, platelet-rich plasma gel, platelet concentrate, and blood plasma therapy — into the soft tissues or around an injury. This treatment has been used successfully in treating certain injuries and conditions. PRP is a blood derivative that contains a more-concentrated level of platelets than does ordinary blood and is enriched with tissue growth factors that can help heal ligaments and tendons. It is used to treat such soft tissue injuries as tendinopathy, acute and chronic muscle strain, muscle fibrosis, ligament sprains, and joint injuries or conditions such as arthritis, arthrofibrosis, articular cartilage defects, injury to the knee meniscus, and joint inflammation. PRP is also used to heal chronic wounds to the skin and to regenerate the bone structures of teeth and the jaw. It is being used in major hospitals to stimulate red blood cell growth in patients with anemia or kidney failure. In short, PRP regenerates tissue and stimulates the healing process.

PRP has been used for years in surgical applications, in orthopedics to heal bone, and to seal and heal wounds. When we injure ourselves — for instance, by getting a cut — the wound bleeds. Once blood makes contact with the injured tissue, proteins break the platelets open and deliver biochemical components that form a clot. The chemicals in that clot, specifically growth factors that are specialized by the type of tissue in the body, go to work to heal the wound. Once the clot is in place, the inflammation response begins, which drives white blood cells and stem cells to the area. Tissue is then regenerated, new blood vessels are formed, and new tissue bonds with mature tissue. Gradually, the injured tissue returns to normal.

PRP therapy works by extracting from blood the growth factors, stem cells, and fibroblasts that support the healing and tissue growth process and then transplanting them directly to the injured site or joint to promote healing. In PRP treatment, blood is taken from the patient and is processed in a centrifuge to separate the PRP from other components in the blood. This use of blood is called autologous because it is taken from and used in the same person. So there is no concern that someone using this method could pick up an infection or disease from another person. The PRP is then injected into the injured area. The entire process of removing the blood and extracting the PRP typically takes just fifteen to twenty minutes.

A typical treatment begins with the identification of the injured tissue using real-time ultrasound guidance or real-time fluoroscopy (a computerized X-ray machine that lets you look into the body from every direction). Then the physician sterilizes the skin and anesthetizes (numbs) the region so that the treatment is painless. Next, under direct imaging, the physician transplants the platelet tissue into the damaged area. Sometimes, the physician adds calcium and thrombin (scaffold material) as needed to enhance the tissue matrix and support the growth of new tissue.

Typically, a person undergoing this treatment receives injections once every four weeks. The average number of treatments needed to heal an injury is between four and seven. Patients usually feel improvement by the third or fourth treatment, sometimes sooner.

The risks with PRP treatment are minimal. It is common to feel pain and have increased swelling for three to five days after the treatment. Infection risk is minimal (1 in 50,000). To minimize infection risk further, an antibiotic is sometimes added to the treatment. An allergic reaction to local anesthetic or an injury to an adjacent structure can occur as in any procedure, so it is important that you be treated by a trained and skilled clinician who is prepared for any adverse events. Although rare, pain or dysfunction can worsen for a few weeks if the inflammation is intense.

Let me tell you about one patient in particular. Ed is a fifty-year-old man with severe hip arthritis. He was told by two orthopedists that he needed a hip replacement. His pain was severe—consistently a seven on a scale of one to ten—and he could not cross his legs. He enjoyed being active—running and playing basketball—but the pain was becoming too much to bear. After only four PRP treatments, his pain dropped to zero. He was back playing basketball and could cross his legs without pain. He now gets a booster shot once every six months and is living a normal, healthy life.

PRP therapy has been used to treat hundreds of patients like Ed whose orthopedic problems ranged from arthritis to tendinitis. The treatment alleviated the pain and repaired the injuries in more than 90 percent of the cases. PRP is safe, less expensive than surgery, and very effective. The knowledge base surrounding PRP is increasing daily, and soon it may be used to repair organ injuries, neurological injuries, disc conditions, and degeneration of the joints.

GROWTH FACTORS

The use of growth factors is a method of promoting healing without the inflammatory cascade that has long been used to treat various illnesses. Growth factors are hormone like and can have a powerful effect on individual cell proliferation. These unique proteins are made by the affected cell or by distant unrelated cells. Following are a few examples.

- Erythropoietin is a growth factor that primarily stimulates the proliferation of red blood cells. This growth factor has saved many lives by treating the anemia associated with chronic renal failure, cancer treated with chemotherapy, and AIDS.

- Filgrastim works primarily within the bone marrow to stimulate neutrophil—a type of white blood cell—proliferation. This can be used to treat certain types of leukemia and individuals with cancer whose bone marrow function is suppressed by chemotherapy.

- Insulin-like growth factor (IGF-1), platelet-derived growth factor (PDGF), and transforming growth factor (TGF), all found in your blood, can also be used to heal injuries not responding to the usual remedies. Injecting ones' own blood can make even normal tendons stronger. In one study of 28 patients with chronic tennis elbow, total resolution of the subjects' chronic pain, even with vigorous activity, was achieved in 23 of the patients after one to three injections (Edwards 2003). Another option is to isolate a single growth factor in a laboratory and inject it into injured tendons or ligaments.

- Simple glucose has been used as a growth factor stimulant.

Just as prolotherapy harnesses the beneficial effects of the body's natural inflammatory cascade, so is it with growth factors. With prolotherapy, the stimulation of a cells ability to produce growth factors is initiated by an injection of a simple solution designed to trigger that response.

Stem Cell Injections

A treatment similar to PRP therapies is the injection of stem cells into damaged tissue, particularly torn ligaments and tendons and worn joint structures. Stem cells—adult stem cells, not embryonic or umbilical stem cells—are undifferentiated primal cells that exist in the bone marrow and are still capable of becoming a diverse array of tissue cells, such as tendon, ligament, muscle, nerve, and organ cells. This treatment option is well suited to treating injuries or conditions that may otherwise require surgery.

Stem cell injections are used to treat

- Fractures that have failed to heal;
- Joint cartilage problems;
- Partial tears of tendons, ligaments, or muscles;
- Chronic bursitis; and
- Avascular necrosis of the bone.

Stem cells are also used to treat diseases or conditions that cause the degeneration of tissue, although this is primarily happening only in Europe at this time.

This option is more expensive than any of the other injection therapies, primarily because of the complexity of retrieving stem cells from your body and then growing them in a laboratory. It is therefore generally reserved for more severe injuries or those injuries that do not respond to prolotherapy or other treatments. Regenexx is one of the companies pioneering the use of stem cells as an alternative to surgery. A description of their process for the stem cell procedure follows.

Stem cells are most commonly harvested from the marrow of a person's hipbone. This process can be painful, so the area is numbed. The process generally takes twenty to forty minutes. PRP is also taken from your blood so that growth factors can be used to grow more stem cells in a culture. The process of growing stem cells in the lab typically takes a few weeks. The goal is to be able to inject more than a million stem cells into the affected area. If any cells are not used, they can be stored (frozen cryogenically) for later use. While the cells are being grown, they are given certain chemical cues (based on the problem being treated) so that they know what types of tissue to build once they are injected.

Once the stem cells are grown, they are injected into the soft tissue with the expectation that they will go to the injured site and promote repair. After the treatment, patients are asked to use an at-home infrared device to promote the further growth of stem cells. In addition, patients take supplements to support healing and the health of the joints.

Patients may experience results in one to three months, but the repair process may take as long as nine months. Because the procedure is neither invasive nor debilitating, most people can return to limited activity right away and gradually increase their activity over time.

Despite its value, there is a major concern about this procedure. The price: It costs between $7,000 and $8,500, and many insurance companies do not currently cover the expense.

As you've learned, several types of regenerative injection therapies are available to relieve joint and back pain and injuries. It is my belief that prolotherapy is the best option for many people. It is more effective than dry needling because it causes greater delivery of growth factors, a beneficial and inflamatory reaction, and it is less expensive than PRP therapy and substantially less expensive than stem cell therapy. The next chapter explores prolotherapy in more detail to help you determine whether it is the right choice for you.

Chapter 8

The Prolotherapy Path

Sam was a really good racquetball player. Winning matches against the best players in his area, he wasn't ready to quit playing any time soon. He headed to the courts every day after work to relieve his stress. Eventually, however, it became difficult for him to play because his knees would swell and become painful, worsening after each game. When it took a significant amount of time and energy to recover after a match, Sam realized that it was time to seek the help of a medical professional. Unfortunately, X-rays and an MRI revealed that he had advancing osteoarthritis.

Deciding which doctor to visit was a challenge. Sam had actually heard of prolotherapy, but he scheduled an appointment with a primary care physician who had treated his sports related injuries before. The two discussed his progressively worsening knee injury, after which Sam decided—with his doctor's encouragement—that a visit to my office would be beneficial. Because this was Sam's first experience with prolotherapy, he had many questions about the treatment and the process.

At this point, you may be just as curious as Sam was about this treatment with the odd-sounding name. So far, I've described the basics of how prolotherapy works and why it is an effective treatment. Now let me answer the other questions you may have by describing prolotherapy treatment in detail. (Note that I conclude the book with a chapter on how prolotherapy can treat specific conditions. Before we get to that point, however, it's best that you understand exactly what the treatment involves.)

Is Prolotherapy Right for You?

Are you wondering if prolotherapy is right for you? To help you make that determination, take a few minutes to read the following list of questions and answer them honestly. This list was adapted from William J. Faber and Morton Walker's book *Pain, Pain Go Away* (2007):

- Do you use a brace, splint, or supportive strapping for an uncomfortable body part on a regular basis?
- Do you have to frequently change position when lying down because of pain, pressure, or other discomfort?
- Have you ever had synovitis, tendinitis, or another musculoskeletal problem for more than six weeks?
- Have you undergone surgery for the removal of discs, menisci, or other structures and yet still have pain?
- Do you have trouble sleeping or feel pain when you try to get out of bed?
- Do you lack endurance that you once had because of your joint pain?
- Do you experience swelling or body aches after normal exercise?
- Aside from no-impact exercise like biking or swimming, does your joint pain lessen when you are at rest but worsen after exercise?

- Can you stand, sit, or walk for only a short amount of time before you have to change position because of discomfort?

- Have you undergone cortisone or nerve injections for pain but only had temporary relief in the affected area?

- Have you undergone surgery for the correction of tendons, hip replacement, ligaments, carpal tunnel syndrome, spinal fusion or pinning, herniated disc, fractures, chronic joint dislocation, or other related surgery, but you still experience pain?

- Do you take anti-inflammatory drugs, such as aspirin, naproxen, or others, for pain, acute or chronic?

- Do you experience joint stiffness, aching, and inflammation?

- Do you struggle to get out of a chair, walk down the stairs, or roll over in bed?

- Do your painful joints make grinding, popping, clicking, or snapping sounds?

- Have options such as chiropractic adjustments, acupuncture, reflexology, and other bodywork, provided only temporary relief from the pain?

The more times you were able to answer yes, the greater the chance that prolotherapy is exactly what you have been looking for. Even if you answered yes to only one question in that list, prolotherapy may be able to offer relief. Of course, no treatment works for all conditions all the time, and prolotherapy is no different. It is not a cure all, and for some it may not be a good alternative to other more invasive treatment options. But it is a safe, simple, and effective way to resolve complex sprains and other soft tissue injuries.

If you determine that prolotherapy seems like the answer you have been looking for, then you must locate a physician who offers prolotherapy (see the material in appendix A for information on finding a physician in your area). The list of doctors who are using prolotherapy is growing rapidly as more professionals are seeing both the long-term and the short-term benefits and relief this treatment provides.

A Prolotherapy Session and the Typical Response

If you did not read the introduction to prolotherapy in the previous chapter, please do so. It is important that you understand how and why it works before exploring it further as a treatment option. The important thing to keep in mind is that it utilizes your body's natural healing response to regenerate healthy tissue in your tendons and ligaments (refer to the discussion of the healing process in chapter 1).

Before you begin prolotherapy, you should be fully evaluated by your doctor. This is necessary to ensure that your body is healthy enough to recover completely from the treatments and inflammation. As I have stressed in other chapters, it is always important that you share your complete medical history with any doctor so that he or she can determine the best course of action for you. Though prolotherapy is low-risk and has few side effects, it is not for everyone. Providing your doctor with the necessary information not only protects you from receiving poor health advice but also gives you a better chance of healing fully and correctly.

I outlined the typical path I take before arriving at prolotherapy as a treatment in chapter 6, figure 6.1. Obviously, if a patient is injured, we must determine if there was a bone fracture or if there is a severe tear in a ligament or tendon. But if it seems that the injury is primarily a sprain of a ligament or a case of tendinitis, I will likely recommend trying prolotherapy to heal the injury.

An actual prolotherapy treatment is fairly simple. You enter the exam room and the doctor examines the area of injury. Then he or she prepares the site of the injections by disinfecting the skin. Depending on where the injury is, you may be asked to sit during the procedure or lie down. To ease the process, the doctor will likely ice the area where the injections are to be made, or possibly use ethyl chloride to make the area very cold.

Some doctors use an anesthetic, but many do not because the injections cause little discomfort. If you happen to have a needle phobia, your doctor may give you mild sedation to calm your nerves or relax you. Some doctors may even use general anesthesia for the procedure, but this is not necessary. It also adds greatly to the cost of the treatment and comes with all of the usual risks of anesthesia. Once these steps have been taken, you are ready to receive the injections.

In many cases, the doctor manually identifies the ligament or tendon, manipulating the area to identify the best location for the injection. Some doctors use imaging technology, such as ultrasound or fluoroscopy, to guide the needle to the best injection site. This is not an absolute necessity, but in some cases, it can make the treatment more precise. Once the best location is found, the doctor gives the first injection. He or she then continues with a series of injections. The exact number of injections is usually determined by the size of the structure being treated and the extent of the injury. On average, you should expect to receive a dozen injections or so. The process is typically quite fast, particularly after the first treatment.

After your first few prolotherapy sessions, it is unlikely that you will want to start using your injured joint immediately. There will be some residual, but short-term pain and stiffness. The duration of discomfort depends on the severity of the injury. But after a few days, the initial stiffness should begin to wear off. After each subsequent treatment, there should be a noticeable difference with regard to the level of the original pain or discomfort that led you to seek prolotherapy.

I give my patients five general instructions at each visit:

1. Add glucosamine and chondroitin supplements to their diets (as discussed in chapter 5).
2. Do not take any anti-inflammatory medications, such as Advil, aspirin, or naproxen. Tylenol is acceptable.
3. Do not keep the joint completely immobile, but do not do any activity that aggravates the pain of the injured joint. Activities will slowly be reintroduced as the healing occurs.

4. Increase the blood flow to the affected area by applying heat and undergoing physical therapy if possible.

5. If you smoke, stop. Keep your blood sugar, blood pressure, and cholesterol under good control.

Frequency and Duration of Treatments

Sam wondered how long his overall treatment would last. Losing too much time on the court would really affect his playing ability. Would one session heal the injured places in his knee? Or would he have to come in on a weekly basis?

The average course of prolotherapy, according to various studies, involves four to six treatments over a period of a few months. Every person and every injury is different, however, so the number of treatments varies accordingly. The factors that determine the length of the course of prolotherapy treatment are listed next as they relate to the person, type of injury, and duration of injury.

The person injured

- How healthy is the individual aside from the injury?
- How willing is the individual to follow the directions involved with the treatment (rest, rehab, etc.)?
- How available is the individual to schedule follow-up appointments, as well as other necessary appointments?
- Are other injuries or conditions affecting the person at the same time?

The type of injury

- How severe is the injury?
- How many individual muscles, tendons, or ligaments are affected?
- What type of action was taken with the injury when it first occurred?

- Can the location of the injury be easily determined or is it a combination of multiple injuries?

The duration of the injury

- How long ago did the injury happen?
- How quickly was the injury dealt with?
- Have other things (such as surgery) caused the injury to worsen over time?

The less severe the injury, the fewer number of prolotherapy treatments needed. There is no magical number that works for everyone seeking relief. In some cases, only two treatments may be necessary. In other cases, treatment might continue for several months, depending on the degree of improvement experienced after each treatment. This is particularly the case when a person has a physical condition that results in consistent reinjury or restressing of a particular area. Only the prolotherapist, with the patient's full agreement, can make these decisions.

Time is needed between each treatment for the body to complete its healing task. There must be sufficient time for the inflammation to occur, for the soft tissue to heal and rejuvenate, and for the inflammation to resolve. Having prolotherapy treatments too close together may be ineffective. Sam, for example, received six injections over the course of six months, going in for an appointment about once a month.

Most treatments are scheduled once every two weeks to once every six weeks. After a round of four to six treatments, each including multiple injections, the physician reevaluates, along with the patient, to determine whether the injury has sufficiently healed or the condition has been resolved to the patient's satisfaction. Is there less pain? Has mobility improved? Do you feel better overall? The answers to these questions decide how treatment continues. If there is noted improvement, the time between treatments may be lengthened. If the pain seems to have been alleviated, the physician might not recommend more prolotherapy treatments.

There are times when the course of treatment ends but the patient is still experiencing pain. Even if the pain intensity is moderate to low, it indicates there may be more to be done for that person to become pain free. For some patients, a realistic goal is a substantive reduction in pain intensity (e.g., greater than 50 percent), which may be sufficient to improve quality of life and function. What then? Sam's case is a good illustration. After a series of injections and a few months had passed, Sam was playing racquetball regularly; but he continued to have a small amount of pain each time the game ended. I felt that additional prolotherapy treatments, as well as other injections, would help Sam. I decided to use hyaluronic acid (Synvisc) in a series of three injections. (Synvisc is described in more detail later in the chapter.) This provided complete relief for Sam, even when he played several racquetball games in a row. It is important to understand that total pain relief in many cases may not be possible. However, a substantial reduction in intensity can often be achieved.

During prolotherapy, a patient can enhance his or her body's response to the treatment by remaining physically active. Even if it is just physical therapy, massages, or stretching, any amount of movement that helps increase the blood flow assists in what the prolotherapy itself is doing. Immobilization is not healthy for the body—it can cause a build up in fatty tissue around the injury as well as increase stress on the areas surrounding the injury, which could possibly increase the pain. For these reasons, movement throughout the healing process is essential.

> A patient can enhance his or her body's response to the treatment by remaining physically active.

In Sam's case, as long as the inflammation had gone down enough so that movement was possible, he was able to play short games of racquetball while he was healing between sessions, and the exercise was actually beneficial for his recovery. However, once osteoarthritis is advanced, as with Sam, it is best to avoid exercise on hard surfaces. Sam has since taken up cycling.

Trusting your body is the way to know the right time and the right amount of physical activity for you. If it is too painful to walk, just stretch. If you are unable to find any exercises that seem comfortable, a trip to a physical therapist or a chiropractor might be in order. These doctors are able to help you using simple movements to increase the blood flow. Decisions about the length of treatment or rehabilitation should be made with your prolotherapist. As time passes and healing begins, your physician should be able to assess how much rehabilitation you need, if any. Just remember to keep moving between injections — it is the best thing you can do for your body.

Injection Components

Prolotherapists use several common substances to produce a safe inflammatory response in your body's soft tissues. These include:

- Concentrated dextrose (yes, sugar!),
- Glycerin/glycerol (a sweet syrupy liquid that provides lubrication and facilitates the injection process),
- Sodium morrhuate (a mixture of sodium salts and cod liver oil),
- Phenol (an antiseptic used to prevent the growth of bacteria), or
- Lidocaine (a local anesthetic).

Although these components are used in a variety of combinations, they all serve the same purpose — to strengthen ligaments and tendons.

The injectants are mildly irritating and thus stimulate a low-grade inflammatory response. Over time, the once lax structures tighten because they are receiving healing stimuli. It's as though you have injected new resilance into a lax rubber band. Instead of completely replacing the rubber band, or surgically changing its structure, these injections bring strength back to the rubber band (that is, your tendon or ligament). Even fibrous connective tissue surrounding cartilage can be renewed and strengthened. Growth in ligaments and tendons has been directly demonstrated in laboratory experiments and in animal studies particularly with repeated injections (Liu, 1983; Maynard, 1985; Dorman, 1991). Another contributing mechanism to pain relief may be interruption of pain signals through sensory nerve endings.

In addition to using the listed substances to create an inflammatory response, hyaluronic acid, the major component of synovial fluid (the fluid in our joints), is often used to treat osteoarthritis in the knees. I use a product called Synvisc. It works by increasing the synovial fluid and thereby cushioning and lubricating the joint.

Important Note: You should not undergo prolotherapy if you are allergic to any of the primary substances in the injections (see the contraindications section later in the chapter). That said, however, many different solutions can be used in the prolotherapy process, and if you are allergic to one substance, another may be an effective substitute. It is absolutely critical that you discuss your allergies with your prolotherapist before beginning treatment.

THE HEALING POWER OF GLUCOSE (SUGAR)

As mentioned in chapter 7, glucose can be used to stimulate the production of growth factors. Evidence of the ability of glucose to treat osteoarthritis was revealed in a double-blind placebo-controlled study conducted on patients with knee osteoarthritis (Reeves 2000). Three injections of a 10 percent glucose solution were given over a four-month period into 111 knees. The patients had complained of knee pain for more than eight years and had less than 3 mm of articular cartilage left in their knees. This extremely inexpensive and safe treatment resulted in a 35 percent decrease in pain and a 45 percent improvement in swelling. Even the patients' range of motion improved. These results with glucose were far superior to the placebo solution. With this treatment, as with prolotherapy, the knee is treated in a natural manner. The only way to increase the growth factors locally, where they are needed, is to inject the glucose into the injured area.

How Long Before You Feel Relief

Patients sometimes become frustrated when their pain is not markedly improved after a few sessions. Especially when multiple injuries are involved, I often tell patients about "the man who sat on three nails." This man went to a doctor to see if he could determine the cause of the pain. The doctor examined him, and noticing the most prominent nail, removed it. Thinking this to be the cause of all the pain, the doctor assured the patient that he was now cured. The patient happily left the office satisfied that the cause of his torment had been removed.

Later on, however, when he attempted to sit down, the man again experienced severe pain. He returned to the physician's office, angry that he had paid good money to have his pain eliminated only to find it unresolved. Upon reexamining the patient, the doctor found another less-obvious nail, and he removed it. Now, surely, the pain would be resolved, thought the patient, and he left satisfied.

Once again, however, when the patient attempted to sit down, he experienced pain. But this time, he noticed that the pain was less severe and more localized than before. Nonetheless, he was still unable to sit. It was not until the third and last nail was removed that the patient experienced true relief.

This simple metaphor helps patients understand that their pain may have multiple components and may therefore require reexamination and different treatments before a total resolution can occur.

So it is with multiple injuries. Complete relief is often not experienced until all the generators of pain are removed. The process of eliminating pain from long-standing multiple injuries can sometimes be slower and more painstaking than the patient hopes. As the injections heal one spot at a time, it is easier for your prolotherapist to directly pinpoint the more hidden areas of injury. One pain at a time, you will begin to feel relief and strength being restored to your body. Even with more recent or localized injuries, there is no one clear course of treatment. Prolotherapists have no chart they can refer to that says ankle sprains take this many injections and chronic back injuries take that many injections. The course of treatment differs for each individual and each individual injury. The best your prolotherapist can do is give you a ballpark estimation, based on his or her previous experience and research.

In some cases, a patient experiences immediate improvement after the first injection. The injured person is able to move and use the tendon or ligament as soon as the swelling goes down. The most common result, though, is significant improvement after a round of sessions—three or four or more. At other times, improvements have been slower than expected. In such circumstances, I might decide on another round of treatment, or I might change the injection components to help encourage the healing process.

Improvements can be seen as early as two weeks after the first treatment and healing and relief can be permanent after the last prolotherapy treatment. As time passes, the ligaments and tendons will continue to improve in strength and stability. Once the pain is gone, it should stay that way unless you reinjure yourself. By choosing prolotherapy, you are choosing long-term relief from your pain.

Your doctor will monitor your progress as you continue your course of treatment. If prolotherapy is not working for you, your doctor might suggest stopping treatment.

Limiting Conditions

Some conditions definitely limit the effectiveness of prolotherapy. For instance, at times the osteoarthritis in a joint has advanced to such a degree that alternatives like prolotherapy are unlikely to achieve satisfactory results. In such cases, my patients have been very satisfied with joint replacement surgery. Sometimes, though, due to their fear of surgery, their age, or another illness, patients opt to try prolotherapy even though they understand that the results may only be an improvement in pain level rather than a cure.

Even though prolotherapy can be used on people with the following conditions, it may not be as effective because of other factors involved. These conditions include:

- Heart disease
- Diabetes
- Hypertension
- High blood cholesterol
- Smoking
- Obesity

Most of these limiting conditions can be controlled and managed by living a healthy lifestyle. Some people are more genetically inclined to be affected by serious health issues like obesity and diabetes, but by eating right and exercising, nearly everyone can mitigate the genetic effects on their life. Following good health guidelines and exercising for thirty minutes five times a week enhances your body's ability to fight off diseases. Should you find yourself in need of prolotherapy treatments, a healthy body responds much better to the injections than an unhealthy body. You may feel that you are unable to exercise because a severe injury makes it too painful to exert yourself. If you are in pain, a physical therapist or personal trainer can guide you to exercises that will limit the pain while still allowing you to move and maintain a healthy lifestyle.

The most important thing you can do when receiving prolotherapy is to treat your body right as it attempts to heal. Then the healing process will be quicker and easier.

When Prolotherapy Is Contraindicated

There are times when prolotherapy is not recommended. If persons have the following conditions, or if the following circumstances apply, prolotherapy is not considered a good option (Linetsky et al., in press):

- Allergy to anesthetic solutions
- Allergy to the injectable solutions or their ingredients
- Illness that could lead to infection, or an infection in the area of injection
- Bleeding, coagulation, or anticoagulation disorders
- Phobia of needles
- Neurological disorders or problems, particularly if recent
- Acute arthritis
- Acute bursitis or tendinitis
- Nonreduced subluxations, dislocations, or fractures

Prolotherapy Risks and Side Effects

It's important for you to find relief from the pain that you—or someone you love—have to deal with every day. But in being an advocate for your own health, it's equally important for you to know about any risks and complications that go along with prolotherapy. Although this treatment option is low-risk, as with any medical procedure, it involves some risks. These are usually minor and include:

- *Bruising at the injection site*: This side effect is usually minor and fades in a few days.
- *Stiffness from multiple injections*: This is most likely to occur in the cervical area, lower back, and hip, but it may happen in any joint.
- *Nerve irritation*: Temporary nerve irritation might occur from the irritant solution (dextrose or phenol). The irritant solution helps to proliferate new collagen in ligaments and tendons. Irritation at an injection site is temporary.
- *Worsening pain*: This can occur for several days as part of the inflammation induced for healing.

- *Allergy to injection components or other proliferant agents used*: If this occurs, the formulas can be changed to accommodate nearly every patient. The dextrose solution in no way influences blood sugar levels, so diabetic patients need not worry.

- *Headache*: This side effect can occur either from treatment to the head or neck or simply from stress or anxiety over the procedure.

The side effects and risks of prolotherapy pale in comparison to the risks of surgery. And remember, the long-term positive effects are incomparable. That said, complications do occur with prolotherapy, albeit rarely. In one study, Dagenais et al. (2006) surveyed prolotherapy practitioners from two professional organizations. The survey included questions about side effects and adverse events related to prolotherapy for back and neck pain. A total of 171 practitioners responded to the survey. Respondents had a median of ten years of experience and had given a median of two thousand treatments. The most common side effects reported were pain from injections (70 percent), stiffness (25 percent), and bruising (5 percent). Of 472 adverse events (from approximately 300,000 treatments), 69 required hospitalization and 5 resulted in permanent injury as a result of nerve injury. Overall, pneumothorax (a collapsed lung) was the most commonly reported *serious* complication. It was concluded that adverse events related to prolotherapy for back and neck pain were generally benign and similar in nature to those seen in other spinal injection procedures.

What to Avoid During Prolotherapy

When a tendon or ligament is injured, prostaglandins are released. This initiates vasodilation—that is, widening of the blood vessels to increase blood flow to the injured area and thus begin the healing process. Using a nonsteroidal anti-inflammatory drug (NSAID) prevents the release of prostaglandins, thus decreasing the flow of blood to the site of injury. Because prolotherapy injections purposefully stimulate the inflammatory process to boost the healing process and NSAIDs inhibit the inflammatory process, they should not be used simultaneously; they would simply counteract each other, the NSAIDs stopping inflammation and the prolotherapy promoting it. At best, NSAIDs offer short-term pain relief, but they generally cannot heal an injury.

You should also avoid using cold compresses or ice packs during prolotherapy. Ligaments require good blood circulation to heal; ice packs actually slow down the circulation. So, while placing ice on the swollen area decreases the swelling and the pain, it also hinders the healing process. Many people with sports injuries will immediately place ice on the injury. Except in limb-saving situations, this is not really helpful for the soft tissue in your body that is trying to heal. When working with Sam, for instance, I urged him to keep ice packs far away from his injured knee. Though ice packs are commonly recommended to patients as part of the RICE protocol (refer to chapter 3), I reminded Sam that inflammation was actually needed for his full recovery.

Instead, I instructed him to use warm compresses and other forms of heat (whirlpool, heating pad, warm moist towel, etc.) to aid the prolotherapy process. Heat helps with the pain, the warmth causes muscles to relax, and also gets the blood flowing, which is vitally important. In place of ice packs or medications, Sam used heat compresses and physical therapy. That's why, at his last appointment, he was able to tell me with complete confidence that he was back to his old self—able to play long matches of racquetball pain free, and win!

When Prolotherapy Is a Good Supplemental Therapy

Some conditions that result from injury or disease cannot directly be treated with prolotherapy; these conditions require other forms of intervention including surgery. In some of those cases, however, prolotherapy makes an excellent supplemental therapy to strengthen the support of the injured or compromised area and therefore the overall healing process. Prolotherapy can be used in conjunction with other solutions, such as surgery or physical therapy, when it is necessary to maintain and increase soft tissue strength while rehabilitating other injuries.

For instance, spondylolisthesis is the forward slippage of one vertebra over another. Though prolotherapy does help with many back conditions, prolotherapy alone cannot remedy spondylolisthesis because this condition is not reversible. Nevertheless, prolotherapy injections could be used to strengthen the surrounding tendons, ligaments, and muscles to ensure that the slippage did not worsen.

Ruptured ligaments and tendons present a similar case. A complete rupture of these soft tissues means that the tendon or ligament has torn in two. If the areas are completely separated from each other, prolotherapy will not be able to reconnect them. Therefore, the first step in treatment is surgery to reconnect the two areas that had separated. For example, if someone ruptures the anterior cruciate ligament (ACL) in the left knee, the first thing that needs to be done is to reconnect the ligament sugically. Thereafter, prolotherapy can be brought in to strengthen the ACL and the surrounding ligaments and

> Prolotherapy can be used in conjunction with other solutions, such as surgery or physical therapy, when it is necessary to maintain and increase soft tissue strength while rehabilitating other injuries.

tendons to, hopefully, prevent this complete rupture from occurring again and to ensure the full support and functioning of the knee joint in the long term. As with any surgery involving connective tissues, physical therapy and rehabilitation are important parts of the healing process. Prolotherapy would likewise be a helpful option during the rehabilitation phase.

Prolotherapy is not the correct primary choice for people dealing with certain conditions, but in many cases prolotherapy injections aid and speed up the recovery process. Talk with your surgeon, primary care physician, and prolotherapist to make sure that you are receiving the most complete regimen to help you heal as quickly and as thoroughly as possible. Where prolotherapy isn't the primary and best solution, it is often a good accompaniment to consider.

Combining Treatments with Prolotherapy

Physicians who prescribe prolotherapy as a primary treatment will also recommend other types of treatments to support your overall healing process and to correct any related problems. They will also outline an appropriate regimen of physical activity to support your continued strength and functioning. Generally, prolotherapy can be combined with almost any treatment described in this book, including surgery.

Several types of therapy, for example, can help you overcome stiffness or restore strength to a previously compromised joint. Many times, nothing further than prolotherapy is necessary; however, healing may be given a boost though physical therapy, electrotherapy, acupuncture, yoga, and massage. Before you try any of these on your own, however, always ask your physician which therapy—if any—would be advisable for your condition and how long you should wait after your last prolotherapy session before seeking it. As discussed, this varies from patient to patient, depending on the extent of the injury and the patient's overall condition.

Physical therapy is often recommended concurrently with prolotherapy. Physical therapy can help you maintain movement, increase the strength of muscles to resolve other issues, and solve related problems, such as muscle spasms. The physical therapist may employ electrotherapy to resolve neuromuscular issues. Massage therapy is often recommended when a patient's range of motion is good but there are myofascial pain and muscle spasms that need to be resolved. When a person is experiencing spinal or pelvic pain, chiropractic therapy is typically recommended as a concurrent treatment.

Physical Activity During Treatment and Rehabilitation

Although you may be encouraged to get regular exercise during your treatment, in most cases, simple stretching exercises should be the first step. For carpal tunnel syndrome, for example, you need to proceed with caution. Lifting a pot filled with water from the stove to the sink might remain a challenge until the strength of the muscles in your wrist return. And working at your computer, where your injury might have initiated, likely warrants some changes, either in the position of your chair, table, keyboard or in the use of an arm or wrist rest to prevent continued insult to your newly treated wrist. Talking over these things with your prolotherapist can help ensure you do not injure yourself again or prolong the healing process.

The purpose of physical activity and exercise is to strengthen the muscle areas being used. During prolotherapy, it is best if the patient waits until the pain has lessened or even disappeared before beginning much exercise, which could actually worsen the tendon or ligament injury. Once your physician gives you the okay, you should return slowly to exercise, using physical therapy and rehabilitation to bring strength and tone back to the injured area. No matter how long you have been injured, it is likely that some amount of muscle strength has been lost. So, it is best to slowly rebuild the strength in that muscle to ensure continued health.

When Prolotherapy Can't Help

Although prolotherapy is a very effective treatment option for many types of joint and back injuries or conditions, it cannot remedy some types of joint problems. There are times when the standard of care, even when the recommendation is surgery, is the better option.

In my experience, most cases of plantar faciitis are effectively treated with a steroid injection to the inflamed tendon. If the steroids do not resolve the problem, then prolotherapy has a very good track record of curing the problem without surgery.

Another example is certain forms of arthritis. Rheumatoid arthritis is an inflammatory disease of the joints that causes a thickening of the synovium (the lining of the joint capsule) and cartilage damage. Consequently, increasing inflammation in the area would only worsen the problem. Gout, a disease caused by uric acid being deposited in the tendons, is another form of arthritis that is primarily suffered by men. The body parts most often affected are the feet, especially the big toe. There is much pain and swelling involved in this disease; prolotherapy could exacerbate the problem because it inflames and irritates tissue. The correct treatment is to lower the uric acid level.

Certain diseases related to the immune system (either autoimmune or immunodeficiency diseases) can result in joint pain. For instance, systemic lupus erythematosus, commonly called lupus, is an autoimmune disease. A faulty immune response is triggered, and the body's immune system attacks areas of the body such as organs (heart, lungs, kidneys) and the nervous system. The immune response involves inflammation, so prolotherapy is not appropriate or beneficial.

Every now and then patients come to me requesting prolotherapy for chronic pain syndromes. Because their pain is not generated by a soft tissue injury, I have to tell them that I don't believe they are appropriate candidates for prolotherapy treatment. Jerry is one of those cases.

Jerry was desperate. He had had severe knee pain for two years and was no longer able to work on ships in the Houston Ship Channel. He had seen several specialists, including arthritis specialists and orthopedists. He was told he didn't have rheumatoid arthritis or lupus. Steroid injections into the knee were of no benefit. Narcotic pain medications gave him little relief. Finally a very prominent orthopedic group in Houston decided to perform arthroscopy to his knee to "repair" a torn meniscus. His pain worsened. A second arthroscopy was performed and PRP (platelet rich plasma) was also given to his knees. Still no relief. He had read about prolotherapy in his online research and he wanted to give it a try. But during my evaluation and medical history, Jerry told me that the knee would sometimes swell, even without exercise, and become red and hot. Thinking he may have Lyme disease or other undiagnosed infectious disease, I decided to try an antibiotic instead of prolotherapy. Within a week he called back ecstatic—his knee pain was resolving. Sometimes doctors overlook critical symptoms that could help them accurately diagnose a patient. I could have jumped right in to prolotherapy treatments without taking all of his symptoms into account, but by following the standard of care, I helped my patient much more.

Some types of structural abnormalities leading to compression of nerves or severe arthritis may not be responsive to prolotherapy. Now that you have an understanding of prolotherapy, you can begin to see if you can expect to relieve the pain that you are currently experiencing by choosing this treatment. Is prolotherapy the only solution? No. But more and more people are opting to use it to heal their acute and chronic pains to return them to the life they knew before their injury. Prolotherapy cannot solve every injury; sometimes surgery is required. We explore the pros and cons of surgery in the next chapter.

Chapter 9

Surgery: The Option of Last Resort

Anita worked as a school bus driver. One day, after unloading all the students, she fell down the flight of steps and out the door of the bus. Once the initial shock wore off, Anita realized she had severely injured her neck and lower back. Months of therapy, medication, and chiropractic adjustments did not improve Anita's health; she continued to suffer daily pain. Thinking it her only option, she gladly accepted neck surgery as a way to end her torment. Her neck pain persisted, however, even when the surgeon declared her surgery a success. She consequently refused surgery on her lower back. Years later her chiropractor referred her to me as a last resort.

By the time I saw Anita, she was completely unable to work. She had begun to receive disability checks and wasn't sure that she would ever be able to work again. Her face was nearly expressionless but for her pain. Anita was a middle-aged African-American woman, yet she appeared to be much older, and very tired, from years of carrying the burden of her chronic pain. I began prolotherapy treatments after many in-depth conversations with Anita regarding the risks involved and the likelihood of full recovery.

Anita's improvement was slow, but steady. Seeing her big smile as she neared the end of her treatments was quite a reward. Eventually, Anita returned to work, her neck now healthy and restored. It was not long before she asked me to treat her lower back, which also responded very well to prolotherapy.

Was Anita's neck surgery necessary? It's impossible to say. What we do know is that it didn't solve her pain. We can only wonder how much misery and expense would have been avoided had she received prolotherapy shortly after her injury or before going down the surgical path.

Surgery is often touted as the last great hope for patients in pain, especially those with joint and back pain. Advances in surgical medicine over the past fifty years have made surgery seem an obvious and simple solution for many different types of problems. But surgery is invasive and expensive, comes with a host of risks, and is often used even though it can't actually correct the true problem that is causing a person's pain. Although it is a critical tool in life-threatening situations, surgery is rarely the best option for joint and back soft tissue injuries.

The problem is that many people are told that surgery is their only hope, that it is the last resort, when in reality it isn't.

When Surgery Is Necessary

Although surgery is often recommended for various joint and back problems after other treatments have failed, it isn't the only option left standing. Even if a particular problem, such as a herniated disc or another type of abnormality, exists, that problem is not always the cause of the pain, and it can be corrected using other, more-conservative treatments, such as interventional pain management techniques and minimally invasive modalities.

That said, I am not at all opposed to surgery when it truly is the best option. I have referred a number of patients to a surgeon because I knew that there were no other options for treatment. And surgical methods have been greatly improved over the years, becoming less and less invasive through the use of laparoscopic or endoscopic methods.

Some of the injuries and conditions that typically cannot be corrected without surgery include the following:

- *Ruptured ligaments and tendons*: As mentioned in the previous chapter, a ruptured tendon or ligament is one that has broken in two. In most circumstances, nothing other than surgery can connect the two parts so that the injured tissue can heal. Occasionally, a severely torn tendon or ligament that does not seem to be healing may also require surgery to prevent a full rupture and to heal fully. Prolotherapy can help the healing process after surgery, but it cannot connect the two parts.

- *Spondylolisthesis*: As described earlier, this is a condition that involves one vertebra slipping forward and over the vertebra beneath it. The slipped vertebra is significantly out of alignment with the other vertebra in the spine. This puts substantial pressure on the nerves around the slipped vertebra and causes pain. When spondylolisthesis is the result of a traumatic event, surgery is probably the best option because the rest of the structures of the spine have not changed their function to accommodate the slippage. The surgery is typically spinal fusion combined with other procedures to realign the vertebra, if possible, and to remove any materials that are damaged, impeding correct function of the spine, or constricting the nerves (as described in the next section). However, spondylolisthesis can be congenital (you may be born with it), and in those cases, surgery may not be the best option because other parts of your spine may have adapted to support the misaligned vertebra. Also, in rare cases, spondylolisthesis can be caused by surgeries, particularly laminectomies (see the discussion in the next section).

- *Severe, progressive scoliosis*: Scoliosis is a curvature of the spine. While the spine is naturally curved, the curves caused by scoliosis are in the opposing direction—from left to right. There may only be one curve, referred to as a C curve, or there may be two, referred to as an S curve. Generally, scoliosis is first treated with exercises in minimal cases and a back brace in more severe cases. The back brace attempts to hold the spine in alignment. The hope is that by holding the spine in alignment, over time the curves will straighten out. In severe conditions, scoliosis can place pressure on the soft tissues in the chest and interfere with heart and lung function. When a back brace and exercises do not sufficiently correct the curvature or prevent it from progressing, surgery is often recommended. Typically, it is not recommended unless the curvature progresses past the 40-degree mark.

- *Chronic dislocation*: Although a single dislocation typically won't require surgery, if you have a joint that is easily and repeatedly dislocated or partially dislocated, there may be enough tissue damage to the joint capsule to require surgery. Ligaments may have large enough tears to require surgery to adequately reconnect them and allow them to fully heal, cartilage may need to be repaired, or other aspects of the joint may require surgical repair.

- *Fractured vertebrae*: When the vertebrae in the back have been fractured (typically as a result of trauma), surgery may be required to repair the injured vertebrae and remove tissue or bone fragments that are impinging on the nerves.

- *Severe osteoarthritic deterioration of a joint*: As mentioned previously, in cases of severe deterioration of a joint due to osteoarthritis, total or partial joint replacement is typically the best option in otherwise healthy people.

Types of Joint and Back Surgery

Many different types of back and joint surgeries may be performed, with a variety of possible outcomes. The most common surgeries performed to repair joints or the spine are described next.

Repairing Ruptured Ligaments and Tendons

The method for repairing ruptured tendons or ligaments depends on the type of injury. The process for reconstructing tendon ruptures is very similar to that used for ligament ruptures.

For ligaments, a rupture may occur at the end where it attaches to the bone, or it may occur in the middle. If it occurs at the end and the ligament is generally undamaged otherwise, a surgeon can reconnect the ligament using large stitches or surgical bone staples. The bone and ligament gradually re-fuse as they heal. This is fairly uncommon, however, and typically the ligament must be reconstructed. If the rupture occurs in the middle of the ligament, the surgeon may still be able to stitch the tear back together. Again, though, this is uncommon. Typically, the surgeon has to reconstruct the ligament entirely.

Ligament reconstruction is most commonly done to replace a torn ACL (as mentioned in chapter 8) in the knee. For this surgery, the graft material is taken from one of three sources: the patient's hamstring tendon, the patient's patella tendon, or a donor or cadaver tendon. When the tendon is harvested from the patient's own body, a piece of the bone where the tendon is attached is also taken so that the surgeon can attach bone to bone. This makes the healing process easier and more complete. The graft is then attached to the opposing bones using a variety of attachment devices, depending on the type of graft. The graft customarily attaches to the bone within six to eight weeks.

Arthroplasty (Joint Replacement Surgery)

In cases of severe deterioration of the components of a joint from osteoarthritis or some other degenerative condition, an orthopedic surgeon may recommend total joint replacement. This procedure is most often done for the knees and hips using an artificial joint that is made of metal and plastic. Each year about 435,000 people have a hip or knee replaced. A joint may be cemented into place in people with weak bones or people who are not very active. For people with strong healthy bones and an active lifestyle (typically younger people), the replacement joint is set in place and attached to the bone, and the bone is allowed to grow around it. Replacement joints generally last ten to fifteen years.

Laminectomy

A laminectomy is the removal of the lamina of a vertebra or a section of vertebra. The lamina is a bony plate at the back of each vertebra that protects the spinal column. A laminectomy is usually performed to correct a condition called spinal stenosis, which is a narrowing of the canals in the vertebrae that allow the spinal cord to run through the spine or that allow the nerve roots to exit the spinal column. When narrowing occurs, those nerves can become compressed and cause considerable pain. The canals typically narrow as a result of degeneration of the vertebrae, which often happens with age but may also result from a variety of other medical conditions. For some people, this narrowing never actually compresses the nerves, so there is no problem. For others, it causes severe compression and severe pain. Spinal stenosis most commonly occurs in the lumbar spine (lower back) or the cervical spine (neck); as a result, that is where laminectomies are most often performed. Laminectomies are also frequently performed as part of a discectomy surgery (described later), and they may be done to remove a spinal tumor or to adjust the contour of the spine to correct a deformity.

Newer forms of laminectomies are minimally invasive and involve the removal of just the lamina. As you might expect, the recovery time is substantially reduced and there is little need for other procedures to support or repair the spine. More-invasive or complete forms of the surgery may remove the entire back of the vertebra and the soft tissue around it, which includes the posterior spinal ligament. In these instances, a surgeon might also have to perform spinal fusion to support the spine where substantial amounts of material have been removed. The recovery from minimally invasive laminectomies tends to be more positive and faster than from open laminectomies (see the discussion of open versus minimally invasive surgery).

OPEN VERSUS MINIMALLY INVASIVE SURGERY

Open surgery refers to surgery that requires opening a cavity in the body to perform the surgery. It typically involves making large incisions and cutting through fascia, muscle, and possibly other soft tissues. Because of all the tissue damage from open surgery, recovery can be long and painful and the risks are greater than with minimally invasive surgery.

Minimally invasive surgery refers to surgery that is done using laparoscopic or endoscopic methods. It typically requires two or more very small incisions. A very small video camera is inserted through one of the incisions and the surgeon introduces small instruments through the other incision, with which to actually perform the surgery. The damage to surrounding tissue is minimal, and the risk of infection is greatly lessened. Recovery time is typically much shorter than with open surgery, and the outcomes tend to be better.

Spinal Fusion

Spinal fusion involves a bone graft to the front (anterior), back (posterior), or side (transforaminal) of a vertebral pair (or even multiple vertebrae) to fill an area where material—bone from the vertebrae or the disc—is missing. The bone graft eventually fuses with the vertebrae, usually after six to nine months, securing them together and preventing them from moving. To support the spine while the bone graft heals, a surgeon attaches screws, rods, and cages onto the spine. As part of the spinal fusion procedure, other procedures, such as laminectomy, discectomy, foraminotomy, or facetectomy (all described in this section), may be necessary to remove damaged structures that are constricting nerves or preventing proper spinal alignment.

Spinal fusion is used as a treatment for spondylolisthesis and scoliosis. With scoliosis, the spinal fusion may involve multiple vertebrae (those involved in the curvature) and more instrumentation (rods, screws, cages) to stabilize the spine as the bone grafts fuse and heal. Spinal fusion is also used to treat degenerative disc disease, disc herniation, spinal tumors, vertebral fractures, and deformities of the spine.

Spinal fusion is typically an open surgery, but occasionally it may be done using minimally invasive techniques. A relative new technique called thoracoscopy allows surgeons to access the thoracic spine (the middle part) from the side through the chest wall.

(I discuss why spinal fusion is a leading cause of failed back syndrome later in the chapter.)

Discectomy

A discectomy is the removal of a spinal disc. It is typically done when a disc has herniated or ruptured, and the goal is to remove the tissue that is putting pressure on the spinal cord or the nerve roots, thus causing pain. In some cases, once the disc is removed, the surgeon leaves the space open. Often, though, the surgeon fuses the two surrounding vertebrae together using a bone graft (as described previously).

Discectomies are most often done in the cervical spine (neck) or lumbar spine (lower back). This procedure is typically minimally invasive and is actually done through the front of the neck in the cervical spine and from the back in the lumbar spine. A laminectomy (which was explained earlier in this section) is a necessary part of the lumbar discectomy; because of the different approach, it is not necessary with an anterior cervical discectomy.

Foraminotomy

Neuroforamen are the passageways between the vertebrae that exist on either side of the spine. Nerve roots that extend from the spinal cord run through these passages. When those passages become constricted by deterioration of the vertebrae or the disc that maintains a healthy space between vertebrae, the nerves become constricted too, causing pain. A foraminotomy is a procedure for removing bone from around the neuroforamen to widen the passage and relieve pressure on the nerve roots. A foraminotomy may be performed on people with degenerative disc disease, spinal stenosis, herniated discs, or spinal osteoarthritis, as well as other conditions. It may be paired with other procedures to treat certain conditions.

Misguided Indicators for Surgery

"You need surgery." Despite all the advancements in modern medicine, these words seem to provoke more fear today than ever. Fifteen years ago, around the time I began my private practice in family medicine, people were glad when a diagnosis could be given for their pain and a treatment recommended. If the recommendation was surgery, the response was to schedule it as soon as possible and get it over with. Today, that is no longer the case. Often, the patient refuses surgery.

The reason is simple. Some surgeries, and particularly back surgery, result in too many poor outcomes. Everyone seems to know someone who wishes they had not undergone orthopedic surgery. The average surgeon cannot differentiate between the patient whose pain will be resolved with surgery from the patient whose pain will be made worse. This is one of the weaknesses of back surgery—the results are never guaranteed. So many people receive the surgery even if, like Anita, there may have been other options. What follows is long recovery periods and often more pain and suffering.

Pain: The Misleading Indicator

When we are injured, it can take our bodies a very long time to heal, particularly when we are older or have health conditions that limit the healing process. During that long healing time, we may be in pain from the healing injury. That pain causes us to misuse the injured body part—we favor it, we sit awkwardly to avoid aggravating it, we stop exercising. Unfortunately, all of these actions can quickly lead to a variety of other problems, such as overstressed muscles that tighten and spasm or ligaments and tendons that are weakened from lack of activity or improper functioning of a body part. The original injury may have healed, but new problems have resulted in the meantime. All we know is that we are still in pain, and we assume the pain is from that original injury.

Although some conditions do require surgery, time and time again I, and other doctors like me, have been proven wrong in our assumption that surgery was necessary, particularly when we based our decision on a patient's pain level. Do you remember Freddie from the introduction? He had a herniated disc, and I was sure that he needed surgery. He insisted we try prolotherapy, and it completely resolved his pain. The herniated disc wasn't directly causing his pain. It's highly likely that surgery for the disc would not have resolved Freddie's pain.

Michael was a similar case. He had been injured in a fall two years before coming to see me. He had been changing the lightbulbs in a chandelier at work. To reach the vaulted ceiling, Michael had to stand on a scaffold suspended six feet above the floor. The scaffold broke and Michael fell onto a table, which collapsed under his weight. He hit the ground with his tailbone and right shoulder. This resulted in severe pain to his right shoulder, his lower back, and his tailbone. Shortly after the accident, he underwent surgery on his right shoulder, with significant improvement. The top half of his body was back in working order, but the bottom half was a different story. The pain persisted and was so severe that, when he sat, Michael had to use a doughnut cushion to keep the weight off his tailbone. Even then, he could sit for just half an hour before he would have to stand up and walk around. Bending and lifting were impossible. Even emptying the dishwasher was too much for him. Unfortunately, his workman's compensation insurance company was disputing the lower back/tailbone injury, and he was unable to receive any treatment. Because he was a veteran, he finally sought help at the VA hospital.

After being examined by multiple doctors, Michael was finally shown to have a tailbone fracture. The tip of the tailbone was not in its proper position. The doctors tried to manually reposition the tailbone by relocating the broken bone to its proper position. They did this manually, through his rectum, while he was under anesthesia. Unfortunately, this did not improve his pain. Although surgery to remove the broken bone was one option the surgeons at the VA hospital mentioned to Michael, they discouraged it, owing to the low success rate and high risk of infection they had experienced with other such operations.

The first time I saw Michael, he weighed 316 pounds, having gained more than 100 pounds in the two years after the scaffold accident. He became inactive because of the chronic pain he suffered. He had not returned to his construction work and could not even help with household activities.

The prolotherapy treatment began with injections to the posterior sacroiliac ligament around his low back, sacrum, and tailbone. After four months, Michael was able to sit and walk for much longer periods of time. Most noticeably, he was again doing things around the house to help his family. About this time, Michael won his workman's compensation case, which meant his low back treatment expenses would now be covered by insurance. Because he was still not well, his treating doctor referred him to a surgeon. This surgeon also recommended surgery but gave him a much rosier outlook for recovery than did the VA physicians. Four months earlier, Michael most certainly would have accepted surgery as an attempt to relieve his misery, but now he was finding some relief from prolotherapy. Would that be enough?

During the preauthorization process to approve his surgery, Michael continued to receive prolotherapy. When authorization was finally given, the surgeon scheduled surgery. But because Michael's pain was 90 percent better by that time, he cancelled his surgery. Michael eventually made a full recovery and returned to regular activities. The ability to move and work again also helped Michael return to a normal, healthy weight. What would the result have been with surgery? Although it is impossible to know, I believe there is a good chance that he would be on disability now.

Cases like Michael's and Freddie's are lessons for us to heed. The medical community should always attempt to solve a patient's pain through the most conservative treatment possible before jumping to the surgical option.

The Criteria for Disc Herniation Surgery

Bob had low back pain for years. His story is not all that unusual, and you have probably heard similar tales. After undergoing multiple myelograms (a contrast X-ray using a dye injected into the spinal cavity to highlight the space between the bony structures, offering a better view of the spinal cord and nerve roots) and X-rays, the case for surgery was made on the basis of several herniated discs. On the advice of his orthopedic surgeon, Bob decided to undergo spinal fusion of the vertebrae in his lumbar region. After a long rehabilitation and still more back pain, Bob underwent a second surgery. As a result of these surgeries, he had even less mobility than before. He was prevented from cycling (his favorite sport) and running. And Bob's pain did not diminish—it increased! Had Bob tried more conservative measures before submitting to surgery, he might have been spared the pain and expense and unsuccessful outcomes.

Surgery for herniated discs is very common, and for a long time it has been considered the only option. But there is a root cause for herniated discs, and it is imperative you bear in mind that the pain you are experiencing does not necessarily result from the disc itself. Weakened structures — specifically ligaments — that fail to support the spine should be among the first culprits suspected for the pain.

Think of it this way: Imagine you are using a rubber band to hold together a stack of sticks. The stack will not be held firmly in place if the rubber band you are using has lost its strength and hangs loosely. But use a new, strong rubber band, and the stack holds firmly together. In the case of low back pain, prolotherapy strengthens the support structures — as if restoring the strength of the rubber band — and is thus more likely than surgery to correct the problem, and it is a much-less-risky solution. Remember, the real problem may stem from the inability of weak ligaments to hold the structures in place. The problem might not be the ruptured disc; it might be the surrounding structures that don't hold the disc properly in place.

> The medical community should always attempt to solve a patient's pain through the most conservative treatment possible before jumping to the surgical option.

Bob's problem — weakened ligaments surrounding his discs — could not be detected on X-rays, an MRI, or a CAT scan. Those weakened tissues are exactly what prolotherapy can help remedy, however. Many cases of spinal surgery could be avoided if prolotherapy is first used. If surgery is eventually indicated, the prolotherapy treatment will have increased the strength of the ligaments and tendons. Even postsurgically, prolotherapy can play a very important role, except when irreversible damage has been done, as in Bob's case.

When he reviewed the cost of surgery in the treatment of lumbar disc herniation, Dr. Edward N. Hanley Jr., an orthopedic surgeon, observed in the book *Clinical Efficacy and Outcome in the Diagnosis and Treatment of Low Back Pain* (1992) that individuals with this type of pain

> will undergo many or all of the known diagnostic tests (plain radiographs, CT, MRI, discography, electromyography) for lumbar spine conditions in a fruitless and costly attempt to place them into some sort of category for which there is a surgical treatment. After a substantial expenditure of money and evaluation by a multiplicity of physicians, a fair number of these individuals with low back pain will undergo a laminectomy for bulging disc, a spinal fusion for intervertebral instability or insufficiency, or both. Failure of the procedure (which is predictable) may result in yet more surgery for a recurrent disc [problem], pseudoarthrosis, or just plain persistent pain. All of this started because of well-intentioned physicians who felt forced to place these individuals into the diagnostic category of herniated intervertebral disc — a treatable condition. (126–127)

Time and experience show that Dr. Hanley was right. The medical community and the insurance industry, however, have not come to realize that the criteria for surgery are seriously flawed. Unfortunately, there have been many cases when surgery for injuries such as disc herniation was recommended based solely on the MRI results and because a patient's back pain had not resolved with physical therapy and medicine.

The criteria for back surgery related to disc herniation are more art than science. The following list outlines the criteria that doctors use and explains how each item can easily be an indicator of a totally different problem:

1. *Functionally incapacitating pain in the leg, extending below the knee with nerve root distribution*: This common sign of disc herniation

is also a symptom of ligamental sprain of the sacroiliac (SI) joint. Therefore, if the SI joint is tender and there is a positive to equivocal Patrick's test, the leg pain may not be coming from a herniated disc. A Patrick's test is one in which stress is placed on a joint to determine the presence of sacroiliac disease. As pressure is put on the joint, pain on external rotation of the hip suggests sacroiliitis. A negative Patrick's test, but continued pain from the back through the leg, is a good indication of legitimate disc injury.

2. *Spinal nerve root tension signs (positive straight leg lift) with or without neurological abnormalities, fitting the radiculopathy, which is pain at the root of the nerve*: Severe muscle spasm to the piriformis muscle in the pelvis or to the paravertebral musculature of the lumbar spine can make it painful to lift your leg, making this sign deceptive. Severe muscle spasms commonly accompany back pain.

3. *Failure of clinical improvement after four to eight weeks of conservative therapy*: Most back pain syndromes resolve in this period of time after conservative physical therapy unless the quality of the therapy is poor or the injury to the soft tissue (muscle, tendon, or ligament) is too severe for therapy alone. Insurance disputes can delay therapy many weeks, while symptoms worsen and become intractable, or difficult to resolve. Inadequate conservative treatment, such as physical therapy, is one of the most common reasons for unnecessary surgery. Early and well-designed physical therapy can resolve many injuries. The addition of prolotherapy and/or Myobloc (botulinum toxin, discussed in chapter 6) to the treatment of selected patients experiencing back pain helps distinguish leg pain from neurological causes with severe soft tissue injuries.

4. *Confirming imaging study: abnormal myelogram, CT scan, or MRI, correlated to the physical signs and distribution of the pain*: As

numerous studies have revealed, many normal people without back pain whatsoever have abnormal MRIs. It is therefore possible for a patient to have an abnormality on imaging studies that may correspond to the distribution of pain from a soft tissue injury but may not actually be directly linked to that pain. Misdiagnoses based on MRI findings happen far more often than physicians or patients realize. This is especially true if the physician does not look for any other explanation for the patient's back pain. Because it is possible to have abnormalities without pain, it is also possible to have an abnormal MRI and continued back pain that are unrelated.

So, while there are conditions that warrant surgery for a patient, that decision needs to be made cautiously. Make your decision based on the professional wisdom of your doctor, but also consider seeing a prolotherapist for a second opinion and a possible alternate solution. Sometimes surgery is not the solution, and it can exacerbate the problem rather than solve it.

Failed Back Syndrome

Many people come to see me looking to get relief from chronic back pain that has worsened since back surgery. These patients are considered to have failed back syndrome, also called failed back surgery. Jeff, the chemical plant inspector we met in chapter 4, suffered from failed back syndrome. The term is used to describe those individuals who underwent surgery with the hope of a cure and ended up with chronic pain many times worse than the original pain for which they sought relief. To be fair, some individuals probably injured their back to such a degree that no matter how skilled their surgeon, a great outcome was impossible. This is not a question of the ability of the surgeon who performed the procedure. Instead, it is a critique of how often surgery is chosen to heal back pain when, in reality, it is not the best solution.

Many times, patients should never have surgery in the first place, and their surgery does them great irreversible harm. The statistics in support of that statement are discouraging:

- 20 to 40 percent of patients will not find improvement after surgery.
- 10 percent of patients will experience worse pain.

In other words, up to five out of every ten back surgery patients do not recover well. They experience postsurgical spinal pain. The pain commonly occurs six to twelve weeks after surgery. If there is no improvement within three months, the surgery is deemed unsuccessful. Three months is a long time to live in pain before a surgery is labeled a failure.

Much thought and research has gone into what to do with the ever-increasing numbers of patients with failed back syndrome. At their seventeenth annual meeting in Miami Beach, Florida, in 2006, the American Academy of Pain Medicine invited numerous speakers to discuss options in failed back syndrome. Neurosurgeon Dr. Hubert L. Rosomoff was among those who believed that surgery was greatly overused for back pain. In the 1970s Dr. Rosomoff, as medical director of the Comprehensive Pain and Rehabilitation Center at the University of Miami, had performed many surgeries that he assumed would be beneficial; he began to wonder, however, whether all of those surgeries were really necessary. So he devised an intensive presurgical rehabilitation regimen. His presurgical patients were required to undergo a rehabilitation program for a six-month period before he would even consider surgery. This program resulted in a *99 percent drop* in surgeries.

"Backs don't fail. Doctors do," said Dr. Rosomoff. He argued that failed back syndrome — defined by some as persistent pain after surgery or other interventions — often happens because initial patient evaluations are not complete. He noted that the source of the pain in most cases is not from the spine itself and surrounding nerves but rather from the muscles, tendons, and ligaments that support the anatomy.

Numerous government-sponsored studies have shown that people who receive surgery versus those who do not are almost equally as well off after five years. In many cases, the body heals itself over time. The issue may then be whether you are willing to wait five years to feel better. Or are you willing to risk the pain and failure of surgery? Luckily, you don't have to choose. Prolotherapy is the low-risk solution for you right now.

Problems Associated with Failed Back Syndrome

According to an article by James Zucherman and Jerome Schofferman of St. Mary's Spine Center California, several common spinal problems occur as a result of failed back syndrome. The most common include:

- *Instability*: Unstable mobility associated with ligament laxity
- *Spinal stenosis*
- *Recurrent lumbar disc herniation*: Usually within eighteen months of surgery and occurring at the previously operated site; surgical choices for repair are limited because of a higher risk for complications
- *Missed lesions*: Overlooked pathologic processes or structural lesions during the initial surgery, internal disc disruption (defined later), or stenosis
- *Epidural fibrosis*: A common result of spinal surgery, but not often a cause of pain; if pain does result, a laminectomy or discectomy may be required
- *Arachnoiditis*: Nerve rootlets adhere to each other or to inner walls of the thecal sac, the membrane that surrounds the spinal cord; a painful condition that does not respond well to treatment
- *Reflex sympathetic dystrophy (also called complex regional pain syndrome)*: Identified by pain to touch, burning, changes in skin temperature, and soft tissue atrophy

- *Soft tissue dysfunction*: Discomfort often in the buttock or lumbosacral region, usually relieved by stretching or changing positions; possibly a result of scar tissue formation and shortened spinal ligaments

- *Facet syndrome*: Increased segmental instability; degenerative changes noted on CT scan or X-ray; results from disc settling after discectomy or other procedures

- *Internal disc disruption*: Severe pain cause by inflammatory degradation of the disc; the disc develops a tear that allows the center of the disc (nucleus pulposus) to touch the nerve-rich annulus fibrosis

- *Pseudoarthrosis*: Possibly from root irritation

- *Metallic implants*: Pressure irritation from implants can erode the thecal case; cause fracture where surgical screws compress natural elements; or bunching of ligamentum flavum (elastic tissue adjacent to the vertebrae) near the hooks and rods of the implant

Symptoms may also include dull pain or aching in the back, legs, or both, or a sharp pain that radiates down the legs. Further treatment for failed back syndrome depends on the extent and cause of pain.

Although I have used prolotherapy on patients with failed back syndrome, the injections do not always eliminate the source of their chronic pain. Prolotherapy cannot be used to treat a chronic irritation of the surrounding neural structure, spinal stenosis, or recurrent herniated disc with nerve impingement. For those with failed back syndrome, these side effects need to be taken into consideration before scheduling prolotherapy. Though it is possible to partially relieve the pain from failed back syndrome, it is not as likely that the chronic pain will disappear for good. Interventional pain management modalities may offer patients one other option in this circumstance.

Causes of Failed Surgeries

One of the main reasons pain does not improve after back surgery is failure to identify the true cause of the pain in the first place. Ignorance of soft tissue injuries can result in a lifetime of pain or even an increase in the pain that was there before the surgery.

Even when the surgery is successful in resolving the intended pain, complications from the surgery may result in a new chronic pain syndrome. Often there is also persistent pain from back surgery. This could include irritation of local nerves, recurrent/residual disc herniation, irritation of local neural structures, and spinal root narrowing.

Another much-less-recognized cause of chronic back pain after surgery is the increased strain the surgery causes to nearby structures, including tendons, ligaments, and muscles. When one muscle area, or joint, is stopped from doing its job—as is the case after a surgery—in order to recover, the nearby soft tissue areas are required to work harder. This often causes added stress to those other areas. This pain may occur years after successful surgery that initially resolved the patient's symptoms. Delayed pain, even after the surgeon has deemed the surgery a success, is often related to a soft tissue injury, treatable with prolotherapy and/or trigger point injections. Instability of the back from the surgery may have caused a chronic inflammatory condition for which epidural steroid injections may be of benefit.

Spinal surgery is usually conducted to decompress a pinched nerve root or to stabilize a painful joint. Unfortunately, the surgery is not often able to accomplish more than limiting movement by fusing joints together (spinal fusion) or removing a spinal disc (discectomy). Both of those surgeries are described in more detail earlier in this chapter. The real cause of pain is rarely addressed. Removing a disc herniation may not necessarily remove the pain; and if spinal fusion is conducted in one area, despite multilevel disc degeneration, pain may likely be referred to the next spinal level. This could become a never-ending cycle of failed surgeries and chronic pain being shifted from one area to another.

There is also a high likelihood that scar tissue from the surgery will add more pain. Scar tissue that commonly occurs near the nerve root is called an epidural fibrosis. It even occurs in patients whose spinal surgery for the initial problem was a success. Consequent back or leg pain may arise from adhesions that bind the lumbar nerve root.

Spinal Fusion

Another common reason for failed back syndrome is surgical fusion of the back. The whole idea behind it is simple: If it hurts for you to move, surgery can prevent you from moving. There is similar thinking behind using a neck brace. If significant neck pain accompanies simple movements, a brace can keep you from moving your head. No movement, no pain. The idea with the brace is to use it only for a short time to allow the tendons, ligaments, and muscles to heal. The problem with a fusion, however, is that it is permanent.

A fusion is recommended only for back instability. When the vertebral structures are no longer capable of holding the vertebral bodies in place, they cause pain. This can be visualized in X-rays by allowing the patient to move his neck or lower back in full extension and full flexion while measuring and noting abnormal movements. An abnormal movement would be clearly associated with a ligamentous problem. A spinal fusion would then be recommended: surgically going in to the back and placing titanium rods and screws in strategic places to ensure that the location of the pain is held still.

If your ligaments are overstretched and unable to support your back and are thus the cause of your chronic pain, why would you use titanium rods and screws (certainly warranted for severe scoliosis, fractures of the spine, and spinal tuberculosis) to keep your back in place rather than strengthen the ligaments themselves?

According to surgeon Nathaniel Tindel, coauthor of *I've Got Your Back* (2007),

The controversy isn't very controversial. I think the evidence so far is clear. After looking exhaustively at the research (the studies I've cited, as well as many that I haven't), I have to conclude that, if you have back pain, your chance of getting better with fusion is about the same as your chance of getting better with an effective, nonoperative treatment program. That, in a nutshell, is the most important fact in this book. It's the fact I opened with, it's the fact that is fueling a fight in the medical community, and it's the fact that's most likely to do the largest number of back patients some good. (215)

The saddest cases I see are the ones where a spinal fusion has gone bad. The degree of their pain is difficult to describe; the odds of resolving their chronic pain are slim. It is challenging to heal places in the back that are surrounded by rods and screws, things that were never meant to be a permanent part of the human anatomy. It's discouraging to see these same types of treatments used over and over again.

The System Is Flawed

Since mounting evidence shows that the present approach to chronic back pain does not work, what are the alternatives? Unfortunately, no one is asking that question. Everyone except those paying the hospital bills and those who become disabled by surgery appears to be satisfied with the status quo. The objective for surgeons shouldn't be to see how many surgeries they can perform; instead, their focus should solely be on making each patient well.

According to a 2006 Texas Workers' Compensation Study Status Meeting, sprain accounted for more than half of all injuries resulting in lost days of work. Yet, instead of looking at treatments designed to heal ligament injuries, such as prolotherapy, doctors continue to over-rely on surgery to treat sprains. At the Status Meeting, it was noted that although injury rates had fallen, the cost per claim continued to rise. This also leads to higher indemnity costs to pay the workers for their time off.

Other problem areas recently identified within the Texas Workers' Compensation system include

1. An increase in spinal surgeries within the past decade,
2. An increase in the use of medication,
3. A rise in increasingly expensive claims,
4. A growth in the development of the chronic pain management industry,
5. A large number of musculoskeletal (soft tissue) injuries claims, and
6. A rise in litigation.

Although workers' compensation boards nationwide realize they need better outcomes data to improve the quality of care for the injured worker, they doggedly rely on the same old surgeries and ideas — with, regrettably, the same results.

It is time to change the guidelines and educate the people. The medical community as a whole is inappropriately treating a large majority of our patients' soft tissue injuries. And doctors must play a critical role in identifying and promoting the most effective treatments for all types of injuries and conditions.

WORKERS' COMPENSATION STATISTICS

- Sprains are the most common injury in every major industry sector (U.S. Department of Labor, 2007).
- In 2004, the medical costs for back pain alone in our workers' compensation system were estimated to be $20 to $50 billion annually (Pai and Sundaram, 2004).
- In 2001, losses in days worked and productivity as a result of low back pain were estimated at $28 billion annually (Maetzel and Li, 2002).

Balancing the Benefits and the Risks

Patients assume the surgeries they are being offered for their chronic pain have been thoroughly investigated. They assume that the surgery is likely to benefit their condition with an acceptable risk of injury. Every physician should consider the risk-benefit ratio. That is, the physician should explain to the patient how likely he or she is to be harmed by the surgery versus how likely he or she is to benefit from the surgery. If you are in constant severe pain, you may accept a moderate risk of death or injury. If, however, you are not given accurate information, it is impossible to make an informed decision.

The truth is that physicians often don't know how effective many commonly recommended surgeries are. That's because surgical procedures frequently are introduced into regular use without rigorous study. Surgical procedures rarely are conducted with a placebo control to determine if there is any real benefit. As an example, it is estimated that 500,000 arthroscopies are performed annually for osteoarthritis, at a cost of billions of dollars. Researchers at the Department of Veterans Affairs together with Baylor College of Medicine found in a 2002 study published in the prestigious *New England Journal of Medicine* that patients who received a sham arthroscopy received just as much pain relief as those who underwent the actual arthroscopic surgery. An increasing number of my patients automatically reject surgery, not because of any particular study, but because they have seen too many bad results.

Medicine is an art. It is very difficult to determine the cause of chronic pain. Patients must balance the benefits and the risks. Let's just say that there is a 36 percent chance of a cure (assuming the device itself does not have long-term detrimental effects) and a 10 percent chance of having your life ruined. You must weigh those odds and determine if you should first try other less-risky options. This decision is made more difficult if you are not given all the options. Prolotherapy has a very low risk of harming you when someone well trained does the procedure.

After you consider the cost, risk, and complications of back surgery in particular, you might wonder why anyone would choose back surgery if it is not *wholly* necessary. It is not that surgery is never the correct choice. As I've already discussed, sometimes surgery, though risky, is the best option. There will always be a need for surgery, but only after a more thorough evaluation and treatment aimed at helping the body heal prove not to be enough.

It is important, for you and your family, that you make an educated choice about your pain and how to relieve it. Before you accept "the inevitable" in the form of surgery, explore the possibilities. Surgery is, after all, irreversible, and surgical failures are devastating and life altering. At this point, the medical system focuses on alleviating the pain, not strengthening the structures responsible for the pain. The downhill slide after a failed surgery is fast and includes lessened mobility and increased pain, not only in the original site but also in surrounding areas. When ligaments and tendons remain loose, pain will be referred to other parts of your body. This causes your muscles to go into spasm as they try to realign your support structure. This process creates yet more pain. Though surgery can be effective, and at rare times truly is the best option, there are many risks involved with back and joint surgery. And the knowledge that a complete recovery is not guaranteed should cause anyone to pause before accepting surgery as the best solution. Although there are some risks and a few possible complications with prolotherapy, this alternative treatment is simple and much less painful than surgery.

Chapter 10

How Prolotherapy Can Treat Specific Conditions

Professional athletes train in order to avoid injuries. Playing a sport night after night, though, eventually takes a toll on any body. This was the case for Joe, a professional basketball player in China. He is the team's center and a star player who brings the crowd to their feet with spectacular blocks and shots. He is looking forward to a long career and even possibly playing for the NBA someday. But like many other professional athletes, Joe's future was in jeopardy because of a mid-game mishap.

A few years ago during a game in Korea, Joe was attempting an all-star block when his arm hit the basketball rim; immediately, and painfully, he dislocated his shoulder. With some manipulation from the team trainer, Joe's humerus bone was restored to its proper position. Somehow, pushing through the pain, Joe returned to the court and finished out the game. In fact, he continued to play the rest of the season, but any time Joe exerted himself significantly, the dislocation would occur again. This would happen many times during a game, causing Joe to stop play because of the agony.

As many spectators looked on, Joe would hobble to the sideline, arm dangling uselessly at his side, and the team would have to take a time-out. The trainer would force Joe's shoulder back into position and then the play would continue.

Spending the off-season in the United States, Joe was still working out to keep in shape and began to realize that simple exercises were becoming increasingly painful even when his shoulder would stay in place. When the pain became unbearable and Joe began to seriously worry about the future of his basketball career, he went to an orthopedist. An MRI revealed a rotator cuff tear, and surgery was recommended. Joe was reluctant to agree to an operation, however, having seen firsthand how other players' careers had ended because of poor surgical outcomes. Hoping there was some other less-risky way to ease the pain, Joe searched the Internet to find an alternative solution.

Learning more about prolotherapy, he decided to give it a try. He arrived at my office for a consultation. I gave him a thorough medical examination and reviewed his medical history. I determined that Joe's injury was a perfect candidate for prolotherapy and the treatments began. Because Joe had repeatedly reinjured his shoulder, I told him to expect the treatment process to take some time. After ten treatments, his shoulder felt more stable, and he was able to lift weights in the gym without pain. Though cautious, he returned to playing pickup games around the neighborhood; his shoulder felt great.

Joe has not had a single shoulder dislocation since his prolotherapy treatments ended, and he has returned to his normal activities without restrictions. Now back on the basketball court, he is one of the starting centers in the Chinese professional league. But most important, Joe is able to play pain free. He did his research and realized that prolotherapy was the best solution for his injury.

What about you? How can prolotherapy help heal your injury? In this chapter, I review some conditions that are poorly understood by the medical community and demonstrate how even long-term disability can be treated effectively with prolotherapy. I list specific injuries and how prolotherapy has helped remedy the pain that goes along with each one. Is this an exhaustive list of every pain that has ever been healed by prolotherapy? Absolutely not. But these are the injuries that I see most often. If the pain you are experiencing is not specifically discussed here, does that mean that prolotherapy will not work for you? Not necessarily. This is another reason why seeking out a prolotherapist and going over your physical evaluations and medical history are so important. Let your local physician trained in prolotherapy decide how best to address your pain. Remember, other doctors had solutions for Joe's shoulder injury, but he found the real relief with prolotherapy.

Whiplash Injury

One of the most gratifying injuries to treat is a whiplash injury, also known as postconcussion syndrome. Frequently, after being in a car accident or suffering a head trauma, a person is left with constant or intermittent headaches. Headaches from whiplash injury can be occasional and mild or they can be severe and constant. These headaches are generally the result of tears to the splenis capitis muscle at the base of the skull. The forceful extension of the head forward results in a tear to the tendon. Tears to the fibrous osseous junction, where the tendon attaches to the bone, can result in a referred pain pattern, muscle spasms, and other symptoms. Whiplash injury is also called neck sprain or strain, depending on the severity of the injury. It may also include injury to the intervertebral joints, discs, ligaments, cervical muscles, and nerve roots.

Ollie drove to my office for a routine physical, head pounding. But this was nothing out of the ordinary. She dealt with chronic migraines even though her day-to-day responsibilities could not be ignored because of them. While this sixty-five-year-old woman and I were reviewing her medical history, she described the headaches she had been experiencing throughout her entire adult life. She had seen many physicians as a young woman, and when no remedy could be found, she had learned to accept her condition, taking painkillers daily and muscle relaxants to partially relieve the pain. In other words, Ollie had learned to manage the pain, not really overcome it.

When examining her, I noted tenderness along the left side at the base of Ollie's head, and I asked her if she had ever had a whiplash injury or head trauma. Thinking back, she recalled a horrific car accident from her teenage years: She had been riding around with her friends, a stop sign was ignored, there was a collision, and Ollie was thrown from the car. She was hospitalized for a month with a fractured pelvis and other injuries. During that time, she had severe generalized pain and was receiving narcotic medication for relief. It was also around that time that her headaches began, but she had never before associated that chronic pain with the accident.

After this discussion, I suggested she try prolotherapy for her headaches. Within five treatments, her headaches were gone, and Ollie no longer takes any pain medication. Most of the people that I treat have suffered more recent trauma, but the relief can be just as dramatic. Despite the fact that Ollie's trauma had occurred decades earlier, prolotherapy was successful.

In the case of whiplash injury, patients often experience pain radiating to the front of the head that may be squeezing or throbbing in nature. The muscles along the neck can become very tight. Many people experience dizziness. All of these symptoms can be aggravated by activities that stretch the injured tendon, such as reading or looking down. Frequently, patients find that the pain is so intense, it is impossible to read while looking down at a book; instead, they must bring the book up to eye level.

Whiplash injuries are typically treated with antimigraine medicines, narcotics, muscle relaxants, and anti-inflammatory medications—with little relief. They are difficult to treat because, typically, they involve all three soft tissues: ligaments, tendons, and muscles.

Spending thousands of dollars in physical therapy rarely yields a long-term cure. Few neurologists know what to do with these headaches. If you are unlucky enough to have had an abnormal cervical MRI, you will probably be offered surgery, and you may be desperate enough to agree. After the surgery, your headaches are likely to be compounded by neck pain. Patients who experience this problem go from specialist to specialist in the medical community looking for relief of their chronic headaches. A few people are lucky enough to learn about prolotherapy and find relief.

Whiplash and head trauma injuries are frequently accompanied by neck (cervical) pain. Most often, the injury is to the lower cervical spine where the neck attaches to the thorax. In a serious accident, the neck can be stretched beyond its normal range, tearing a variety of ligaments. As previously described, patients most commonly complain of pain when they bring their chin down to their chest. This pain results from stretching torn ligaments. As the muscles contract to prevent stretching of the injured ligaments, the patient often feels what is described as stiffness. Over time, a severe muscle spasm may develop, further aggravating pain upon movement.

If the head is thrown forcefully from side to side, the levator scapular muscle (which connects to the cervical spine at the top and at vertebrae C3 and C4 and to the scapula, or shoulder blade) also becomes involved. This pain occurs higher in the neck and extends to the upper corner of the scapula. It worsens when the head is turned. If the muscles attached to the cervical spine and scapula are torn, prolotherapy can help resolve the pain. Forceful extension of the head backward may injure the sternocleidomastoid muscle (which connects to the base of your skull on the side toward the back and to your clavicle, so it runs up the side of your neck). Usual treatment options include neck traction, isometric

> Prolotherapy can mend torn areas of soft tissue that have come about because of whiplash.

exercises, ultrasound, massage, and painkillers such as NSAIDs (which were discussed at length in chapter 3).

It can be very frustrating for individuals involved in severe car accidents to be told nothing is wrong with them. Some symptoms might disappear in four to six weeks, while others become chronic. Patients can experience severe, constant headaches and neck pain extending into the shoulder blade and yet have a normal CT scan of the head, MRI of the neck, or X-ray of the shoulder. Patients with these types of injuries are often told, in essence, "to get over it." It is little wonder that many whiplash patients struggle so long that they become depressed.

Prolotherapy can mend these torn areas of soft tissue that result from whiplash. These treatments allow you to live a normal life again, whether that is reading comfortably, driving long distances, or simply having headache-free days.

Shoulder Injury and Dislocation

The shoulder has a wide range of motion and therefore requires a strong joint capsule. The joint capsule is made up of ligaments that hold the humerus bone to the scapula (also known as the shoulder blade or wing bone). This joint is reinforced by the rotator cuff, which is made up of four individual muscles: supraspinatus, infraspinatus, teres minor, and subscapularis. As shown in figure 10.1, they all originate at the shoulder blade and connect to the humerus (upper arm bone).

Tears to the joint capsule result in ligament laxity so that the humerus falls out of its socket. One such example is exactly what happened to Joe, the basketball player. The dislocation had caused a complete tear in the rotator cuff, as seen on the MRI. A few weeks after the prolotherapy treatments ended, Joe returned to my office in a panic. A basketball team had asked him to sign a contract for the next season, but there was one stipulation that troubled him. He was required to have a repeat MRI on the right shoulder. Joe feared that evidence of his rotator cuff tear would prevent him from being signed. I advised him

Figure 10.1: Shoulder Anatomy

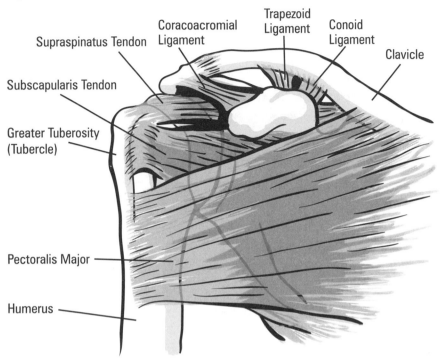

Supraspinatus Tendon

Coracoacromial Ligament

Trapezoid Ligament

Conoid Ligament

Clavicle

Subscapularis Tendon

Greater Tuberosity (Tubercle)

Pectoralis Major

Humerus

to have the MRI done, as requested, and if necessary, I could document his strength and range of motion and hope it would be satisfactory to his new team. The MRI came back normal; the tear was gone. Thanks to prolotherapy, rehabilitation, and rest, there was no evidence on the MRI that an injury had ever occurred in his right shoulder. This was one of the first times I had proof that prolotherapy could heal known tears big enough to be seen on an MRI.

Shoulder injuries are very common in athletes, but unlike Joe's case, many of the injuries occur to the shoulder because the athlete falls on it. Brian was an All-American college baseball shortstop. During one of his games, he attempted a diving catch to his left, becoming horizontal. His left shoulder was driven into the ground and popped out of the socket. Brian hobbled off the field and into the dugout. With great difficulty, the trainer was able to put his shoulder back into place.

Brian was in a lot of pain, and when he visited the team's orthopedist the next day, the doctor wanted him to get an MRI. Because I had treated Brian for a previous injury, he insisted on coming back home to Houston to my office before any other intervention was done. With the future of his baseball career at stake, Brian wanted to put his recovery in the hands of someone he trusted.

Brian was able to move his shoulder, but not without lots of pain. During his treatments, he was restricted to light activity — no baseball playing and definitely no diving catches, no matter how beautifully executed. Eventually, Brian's articular capsule of his left shoulder was fully healed after prolotherapy treatments, and he returned to his college team as their leading batter the very next season. Brian was signed to a minor league team, and he passed an intensive shoulder exam with flying colors. Had Brian agreed to the surgery the orthopedist he saw in the training room repeatedly asked him to consider, the seeds of an arthritic shoulder would have been sown and his career was sure to have been shortened.

Tennis Elbow

Boswell is a skilled dentist whose favorite hobby is playing racquetball. He is one of the best racquetball players in his age group in the United States. After playing a few matches in a row, his right elbow began to hurt, and the pain interfered with his game. It wouldn't go away with the usual rest, pain medication, and physical therapy. Boswell had tennis elbow.

Frustrated with the pain and fearful of losing his place in the local rankings, Boswell knew he didn't want to undergo surgery, and that's when he began to consider prolotherapy. Researching prolotherapy online, he found the nearest prolotherapist — me. Although he had to travel more than an hour each way for treatments, he was committed to the treatment program. I began by treating the tendon of the medial epicondyle. Within three sessions, the back of Boswell's elbow felt almost completely healed. He was ready to go out and play, but I had to convince him that all was not well yet. The tendon of the lateral epicondyle, inside the elbow, took longer to heal, which frustrated Boswell greatly. After all, he was missing multiple tournaments and watching as other players, many of whom he had beaten previously, were walking away with trophies that he felt he deserved. But rest is required to properly heal a torn tendon or ligament. If he tried to play too soon, Boswell risked compounding the torn tendon injury with tendinitis.

The elbows are a common source of chronic pain because they are frequently involved in repetitive activities. Tennis elbow (also known as epicondylitis) is the term given to injuries of the tendon attached to the lateral epicondyle, the end of the humerus bone that connects, via tendons, to the radius in the lower arm (see figure 10.2). In athletes,

Figure 10.2: Elbow Anatomy

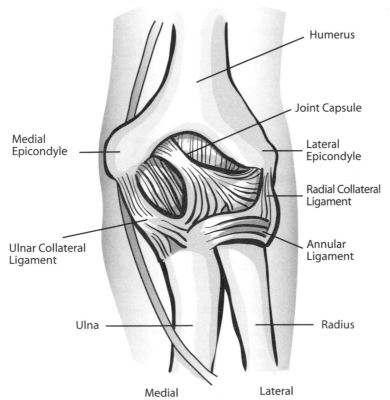

lateral epicondylitis occurs frequently from racquet sports and in workers, from twisting valves or screwdrivers. Most of the time the pain is from tendinitis, and a cortisone injection can be quite effective.

If the pain is not relieved completely after two injections of cortisone, however, prolotherapy should be considered. Tears to the tendon connecting to the lateral epicondyle are slow to heal. Pitchers commonly undergo the "Tommy John surgery" to repair this tendon. A little-used tendon from the wrist is removed and used to reattach the muscle in place of the injured tendon. The outcome can be quite successful, but the procedure contains significant risk. There is no way the replacement tendon can replicate the nerve attachments of the original tendon, which help in spacial orientation. This is of critical importance to the elite athlete.

Injury to the inside of the elbow is referred to as golfer's elbow (also known as medial epicondylitis) and is usually a form of tendinitis. This condition generally responds very well to cortisone injections unless the tendon is torn. A torn tendon calls for prolotherapy.

Knee Injury

A stable knee requires healthy ligaments (cruciate ligaments and collateral ligaments) and muscles. The cruciate ligaments are so called because they form a cross. The anterior cruciate ligament (ACL, which you read about in chapter 8) is located toward the front of the knee, while the posterior cruciate ligament (PCL) is located toward the rear of the knee. As you can see in figure 10.3, the collateral ligaments include the medial collateral ligament (MCL) and the lateral collateral ligament (LCL). These terms are familiar to athletes, active people, and sports fans alike—they are very common points of injury.

The medial and lateral collateral ligaments help maintain knee stability with side-to-side movements. The anterior and posterior cruciate ligaments add stability to the knee to prevent abnormal back and forth movements. With severe blows, it is common that the ligaments are torn completely, thus requiring surgical repair. If only a sprain has

Figure 10.3: Ligaments of the Knee Joint

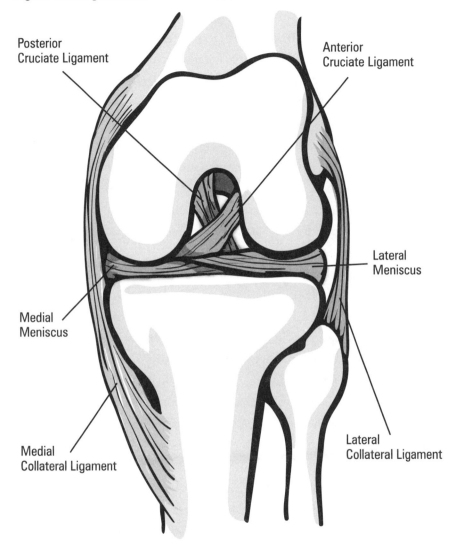

Posterior Cruciate Ligament

Anterior Cruciate Ligament

Lateral Meniscus

Medial Meniscus

Medial Collateral Ligament

Lateral Collateral Ligament

occurred, then prolotherapy is by far the preferred treatment. Surgery to any joint even when necessary and successful is traumatic and hastens the development of arthritis in that joint. Thus, prolotherapy should be the first line of treatment.

Injuries of the ACL may occur from stopping suddenly, slowing down while running, landing from a jump, collision (such as a tackle), or changing direction too quickly. Injuries of the PCL may occur from a blow to the front of the knee, tripping, or pulling or stretching a ligament.

Knee pain can come from a variety of different structures: tendons, ligaments, bursa, and the meniscus. Some injuries are best treated with surgery, some with cortisone, some with prolotherapy. The optimal solution, though, is often a combination of two or three of the different treatments. I have seen patients with such severe knee injuries that surgery was required. After surgery, their pain improved but did not resolve. They would commonly have associated injuries to the medial or lateral collateral ligaments, medial and lateral coronary ligament, and anterior and posterior cruciate ligaments. It is not uncommon for a patient who has undergone successful knee surgery to require treatment for persistent, nagging pain.

Prolotherapy is particularly effective in treating sprains of the medial and lateral collateral ligaments. These injuries are common in football players who are tackled at the knees or in athletes whose sport requires lateral movement, such as in tennis, basketball, and soccer. The pain can be constant but is generally worse with twisting motions to the knee, such as when the foot is planted and the person rotates about the knee.

The knees are commonly affected by osteoarthritis, of course, but that condition is not limited to the knee; it can also occur in other joints, such as fingers or ankles. It is usually necessary to initiate treatment with a cortisone injection to the intra-articular joint capsule to decrease the chronic inflammation. Afterward, three to four prolotherapy sessions are administered. The improvement from prolotherapy is believed to be the result of a regrowth of chondrocytes and increased production of synovial fluid. When the disease process is very advanced and the results unsatisfactory, treatment with hyaluronic acid may be provided. (Recall that in chapter 8 I recommended the product Synvisc for this purpose.) The treatment with prolotherapy significantly improves the outcome, allowing most individuals to return to a more active lifestyle.

I have treated two patients who developed severe osteoarthritis from playing racquetball. Their knees would commonly swell and become painful after a game. Other physicians had recommended surgery despite their relative youth (both were in their fifties). The prolotherapy treatment proved so helpful, they continued to play; however, with the continued repetitive trauma involved in racquetball, they will no doubt require further treatments and possibly even knee replacement.

John used to be an active young adult: He played sports, skied, and lived a fairly physically fit life. As an older adult, running his own business, caring for a growing family, and handling other responsibilities, John settled into a sedate lifestyle. Never one to exercise just for exercise sake, he began to gain a few extra pounds each year. Around the same time that John had his fiftieth birthday bash, he noticed increasing pain in his knee. Now overweight, he made an appointment with his orthopedist and was diagnosed with advanced bilateral knee osteoarthritis. After years of imaging studies and medications, he accepted the orthopedist's recommendation for a total knee replacement.

As a self-employed businessman, John regularly sent in his check to renew his medical insurance policy. When the time came for his physician to preauthorize his knee surgery, however, something had gone wrong, and John was advised that the policy was no longer in effect. Even though his coverage had disappeared, his knee pain did not, but he could no longer afford the option of surgery without insurance. Looking for an alternative that would work for his busy lifestyle as well as his budget, he came across prolotherapy. After eight prolotherapy sessions, John no longer had pain doing the ordinary activities of running his business and living his life. Now he is concentrating on weight loss for more long-lasting pain relief.

Hamstring and Quadriceps Injuries

Other important structures along the knee that are commonly injured include the hamstring and quadriceps tendon attachments. These tendons can be injured by trauma, but more commonly, they occur from exercise. The hamstring and the quadriceps tendons are frequently sprained by going up and down stairs as part of an exercise program. The hamstring tendon primarily begins at the ischium on the back of the leg. (Actually, there are three muscles in the back of the thigh: the semitendinosus, the semimembranosus, and the biceps femoris.) The quadriceps tendon primarily begins along the anterior iliac crest on the front of the thigh (see figure 10.4). Tears here are less common but can nevertheless be very serious.

Mary had injured her hamstring during a cheerleading maneuver. The halftime cheer continued without her as she hobbled to the sidelines and fell into the arms of the trainer. The pain was so great she was unable to put weight on the injured leg. She was seen by two

Figure 10.4: Quadriceps Tendons

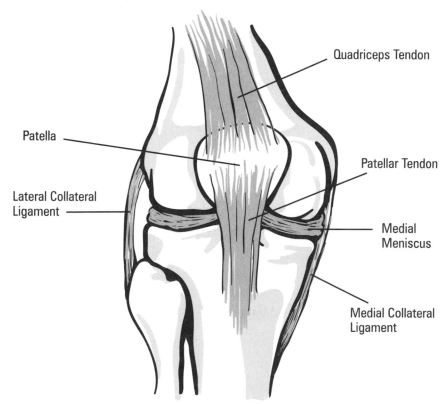

orthopedic specialists and had two MRIs; each revealed a partial tear of her hamstring. Time, rest, anti-inflammatory medication, and physical therapy were prescribed. Meanwhile, Mary used crutches to get around because even the slightest stress on the injured leg caused pain to shoot up and down its length. The physical therapy was excruciatingly painful, and she quit going. Knowing that the cheerleading season was over, Mary wasn't motivated to recover quickly, especially at the cost of increased pain.

After months without improvement, she was told about prolotherapy. Mary came into the office on crutches, still unable to apply any weight to the leg eight months after her injury. With just ten treatments, however, she was pain-free and walking normally. So great was her improvement, in fact, she wanted to know if she could return to gymnastics. Fearful of telling Mary to return to her previous strenuous activities while she still had a partial tear, I ordered a repeat MRI. The radiologist was unable to identify any evidence of the partial tear. She was told to go home and resume all activities as normal. Once again, I had evidence of a tear large enough to be seen on an MRI healed by prolotherapy injections.

Marcus had a different story to tell. He was a professional fighter. Exercising daily was a necessity to keep in top physical shape, not only to survive matches within the ring but also—hopefully—to come out victorious. After a long workout, Marcus would end with sprints up and down the stairway in the back of the gym. He eventually developed pain around his kneecap. Once I evaluated him, I realized that Marcus's pain was not a knee injury but an injury to his quadriceps. Treatment with prolotherapy to the quadriceps tendon attachment around the knee resolved his pain and got him back in the ring. The quadriceps tendon can also be sprained by flexion and extension of the knee during exercise with excessive weight.

Patients are often fearful of returning to their previous activities for fear of reinjury. They often want to know if they need to return periodically for repeat prolotherapy injections to remain pain-free and to prevent the injury from occurring again. I always share this example by way of addressing those concerns: Say you were to cut yourself with a razor blade. You would have to come to the office and have some sutures placed at the site of the laceration. After a week you would return and the sutures would be removed. Thereafter, no further follow-up would be needed; the cut had been healed. It's the same with prolotherapy: If, after a series of treatments, you obtain total relief of the pain while at rest and while exerting your body, then you are healed. No further treatments are needed, and no restrictions are necessary — unless you injure yourself again.

Thoracic Injury

Thoracic vertebral bodies are much less likely to be injured than are cervical or lumbar vertebrae because they are held together much more rigidly, allowing much less mobility. The ribs and their muscles hold the thoracic vertebrae as one unit. Injuries here are likely to result from direct trauma. Significant trauma can result in injury to the points at which the ribs are joined to the vertebral bodies, called the costovertebral junctions. As with other joints, the vertebrae in the spine are joined by ligaments. These ligaments can be strained if stretched beyond their normal range. Direct trauma to the rib cage resulting in injury to the costovertebral junctions can make coughing or twisting painful.

Such injuries commonly occur from car accidents. Injury and chronic pain may also affect the ribs attached to the sternum, which are held together by ligaments. Aside from injuries incurred by trauma, I have also treated ligaments that have been damaged from prying open the chest for open-heart surgery.

The muscles that attach along the thoracic vertebral body, including the trapezius and the rhomboid muscles, respond well to prolotherapy. Treatment is usually directed to where they attach along the scapula and neck. Injuries to these muscles occur most commonly when lifting objects above shoulder height. These kinds of injuries — the type that are sometimes ignored and thought of as just a simple ache or catch—are very treatable using prolotherapy. If the pain remains for more than a couple of days, however, and does not respond to medication or rest, the best option is to seek out a prolotherapist.

Sacroiliac Joint Injury

Painful sacroiliac (SI) joints can usually be relieved by prolotherapy. A typical case of SI joint dysfunction occurred with Patricia, who was working as a cook overseas during Desert Storm. While lifting some heavy trash bags, she felt a sharp severe pain to her lower back. Within a day, it was very painful for her to conduct simple movements, especially bending or sitting. She was unable to work in the kitchen because even the task of moving food from fridge to frying pan was too painful. Patricia experienced pain radiating down her right leg but without significant weakness. She improved very little with rest, medication, and therapy.

After five months, Patricia came home to the United States and made an appointment with me to receive treatment. By then she was desperate to get well and get back in the kitchen, especially because the physicians she had seen previously began to speak of surgery. Although her MRI showed only a bulging disc, nerve compression was suspected because of the pain radiating down her leg. Her pain slowly resolved after prolotherapy to the sacroiliac ligaments of her SI joint as well as surrounding ligaments that were also affecting her posture. After a period of strengthening she was able to return to work, serving up foods while remaining pain-free.

In a study conducted by Galm et al. (1998), 46 of 110 patients with low back pain and sciatica also had SI joint dysfunction. Injuries to the SI joint frequently involve the iliolumbar ligament, the lumbosacral ligament, the sacrotuberous ligament, and the ligaments between the fifth lumbar and first sacral vertebrae. (Figure 10.5 shows all of the ligaments of the SI joint.) These are the same ligaments that were causing

Figure 10.5: Ligaments of the Sacroiliac Joint

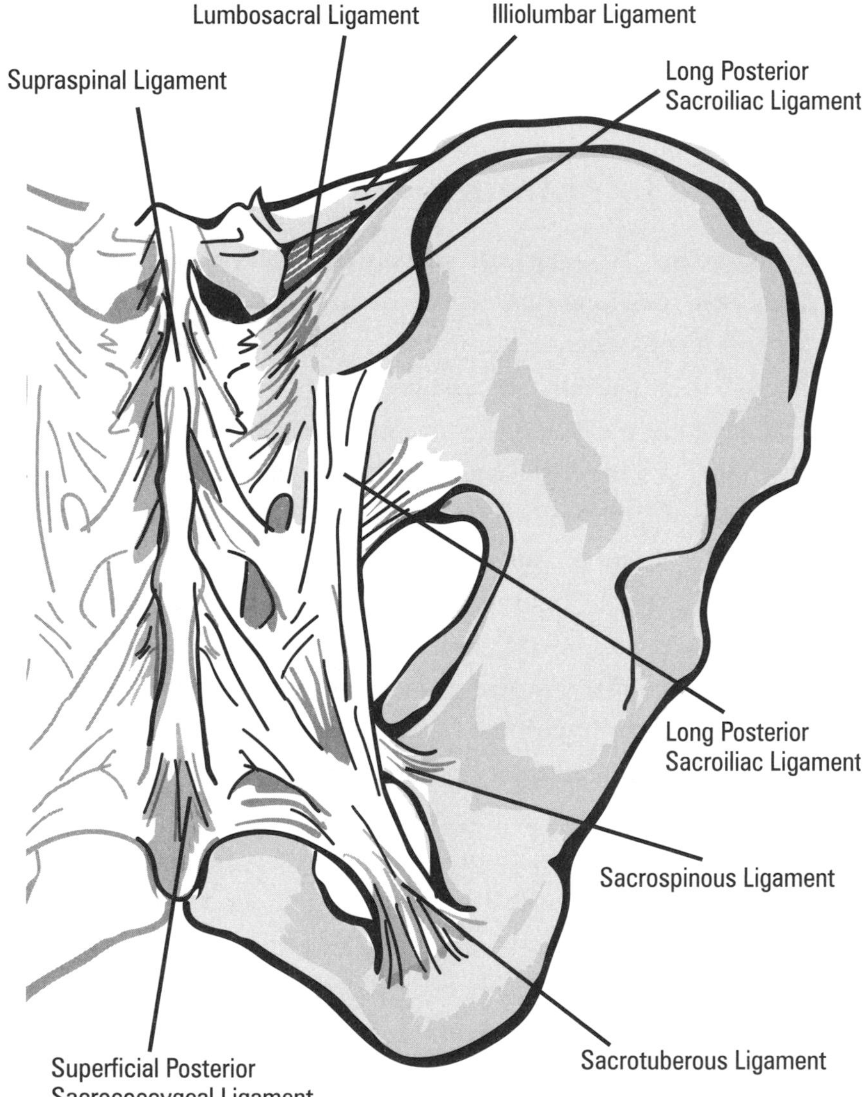

Patricia pain prior to her prolotherapy treatment. Sitting or leaning forward can precipitate pain from the SI joint. Leaning forward to brush your teeth over a sink can be extremely painful when the iliolumbar ligament is involved. Sitting on a bleacher to watch your kids play on a sports field or court can also be quite an ordeal.

Unfortunately, when these ligaments are injured, they commonly refer pain down the leg. This fact results in much misdiagnosis and mistreatment. Good physicians immediately think of nerve involvement and initiate tests to prove it. The referred pain pattern of the sciatic nerve can be very similar. The iliolumbar, sacroiliac, and sacral ligaments are not often examined for pain. Pain in these areas seems to occur more frequently in women. Injury to the SI joint can occur during pregnancy or childbirth or postpartum. This is because these ligaments must become more elastic to allow the pelvis to stretch and make room for the baby's passage. Falls onto the buttocks can also cause disruption of these ligaments.

The SI joint is often ignored because of the difficulty in proving it to be the cause of the pain syndrome. Imaging studies such as X-rays, CT scans, MRIs, and bone scans are unreliable in diagnosing SI joint dysfunction. The diagnosis must be made with the knowledge of the patient's medical history, which should cover such conditions as childbirth or trauma, tenderness along the SI joint, typical referred pain pattern, and such provocative tests results as a positive Patrick's test (discussed in chapter 9).

Because SI joint injuries are often missed as the cause of chronic back pain, they are associated with long-term pain and disability. Benny worked in a factory loading liquor onto trucks. He was originally injured lifting large cases and twisting to stack them onto pallets. Despite being young and strong, Benny found the repetitive bending and lifting to be hard work. One day during a long day of lifting, his back froze; the pain was so severe that he fell to his knees. He had severe low back pain that radiated down his leg. He was unable to obtain relief with physical therapy and medication, including narcotics. He received four epidural steroid injections, which provided temporary relief. Working was still out of the question. Benny's chiropractor suggested he try prolotherapy, but Benny resisted because he "didn't like needles."

Finally, having missed sixteen months of work but being determined to return to his job, Benny overcame his fear of needles and made an appointment with me. His MRI did not show any abnormalities of the lumbar spine or SI joint. His exam, however, was consistent with an SI joint sprain. Several prolotherapy treatments later, his pain was gone. After a period of reconditioning, Benny was thrilled to be able to go back to earning a living. Had he not agreed to have prolotherapy, he would have undergone surgery, which would probably have worsened his condition and resulted in failed back syndrome (see chapter 9). Living his life disabled and on narcotics was no way to live.

Lumbar Injury

Back pain is the condition that I have successfully treated the most with prolotherapy. "I was lifting" or "I was twisting" or "I was bending" are common descriptions of how someone's pain started. It could be the exertion of an excessive amount of weight or simply bending over to pick up a piece of paper. Tears along the supraspinous ligament and intertransverse ligament between the second, third, fourth, and fifth lumbar vertebral bodies generally are felt as pain to the back along the waist. The pain may extend to the leg and buttock. Injuries to the ligaments that join the spine to the sacrum occur frequently. Usually, the injury will be to multiple levels, primarily L4–L5 and L5–S1. The point at which the flexible spine joins the less-flexible sacrum is very susceptible to a ligament sprain.

> Back pain is the condition that I have successfully treated the most with prolotherapy.

Curtis is a strong, tall man in his mid-fifties. He worked hard all his life as a general laborer for the county. Lifting hundred-pound loads was a daily occurrence. One day while loading medical waste into an incinerator, Curtis experienced severe low back pain. Initially, he was barely able to move without pain. After weeks of physical therapy and the aid of pain medications, however, he was able to do simple activities like driving his car and walking from the car to the house without assistance. Being able to return to work was not going to happen any time soon.

Fourteen months after his injury, when physical therapy ceased to offer further relief, Curtis began a regimen of prolotherapy. I worked on the transverse and supraspinous ligaments of his lower lumbar spine in our prolotherapy treatments. After seven treatments, Curtis was free from pain, and although he hadn't yet returned to work, he was feeling hopeful nonetheless. He had stopped all pain medication and had begun a low-intensity workout program that helped him regain strength in the muscles in his back. Several treatments later, he returned to work pain-free, but to this day he continues to be cautious when lifting and moving heavy boxes. Although his back has been healed, if he is going to continue this occupation, improving his strength and flexibility will be important in preventing reinjury.

It is not uncommon for someone to have experienced a back pain that was tolerable for years. Patients often modify their activities or take an analgesic (painkiller) every now and then, avoiding positions known to aggravate the pain. The day comes, however, when the pain is exacerbated by a particular activity and it can no longer be ignored. The support structure of the joint or the lower back finally gives way. Fortunately for these patients, prolotherapy can alleviate the severe pain as well as the mild chronic pain. It is never too late to be treated with prolotherapy.

Hip Pain

Hip pain is similarly a common problem and has many causes, chief among them arthritis, bursitis, tendinitis, referred pain from the back, strain, fracture (most common in patients with osteoporosis), and osteonecrosis—a condition that occurs when blood flow to the bone is restricted (for example, with necrosis of the femoral head). In many cases, rest or stretching will help. In some cases, physical therapy may be required to regain mobility and increase muscle strength. However, when pain persists, evaluation by a prolotherapist is a good choice.

Sacrum/Coccyx

Doctors frequently see patients who have an injury to the lumbar sacral attachment. Injury to the SI joint is less common. Injury to the sacrococcygeal joint is even less common. The more movement a joint has, the more susceptible it is to repetitive injury. The sacrococcygeal joint, just like the thorax, is rigidly held, and therefore, it is usually injured only by direct trauma. The exception is during childbirth, which is a form of trauma. During childbirth, the ligaments become more flexible than usual, and the coccyx may be pushed slightly out of the way as the infant passes through the birth canal. A very large baby, however, may injure the ligaments of the coccyx, resulting in chronic pain for the mother. But an injury to this area is not limited to women.

Other Injuries

Other injuries that I have also treated effectively with prolotherapy include:

- Headache from whiplash
- Migraines resulting from cervical sprain
- Plantar fasciitis
- Musculoskeletal pain
- Some of the pain resulting from scoliosis

The best way to determine whether your injury or pain would respond positively to prolotherapy is to have your doctor examine you and discuss your injury. Each prolotherapist has unique experiences and has seen this type of therapy improve and relieve a variety of conditions. Talk with him or her about your joint or back pain or injury and be assured that there is hope for you to lead a normal healthy life again.

Are you a candidate for prolotherapy? If you have chronic pain or a new injury involving soft tissue, I would say yes. Conditions treated by prolotherapy are many and varied, and I have personally treated most of the joints in the body with it. Every joint and muscle tendon has the potential of benefiting from prolotherapy, and if you choose this treatment, you could avoid surgery, reinjury, and chronic pain. Refer to appendix A to find a prolotherapist in your area and call today to set up your first consultation.

Appendix A

Finding a Prolotherapy Provider

There are approximately 500 doctors across the United States who are certified in practicing prolotherapy. You can use the following resources to find a physician who practices prolotherapy in your area:

American Association of Orthopaedic Medicine (www.aaomed .org): This organization provides information about and educational programs focused on the accurate diagnosis and comprehensive non-surgical treatment of musculoskeletal problems. The website includes a detailed list of doctors who practice prolotherapy.

Journal of Prolotherapy (www.journalofprolotherapy.com): This online journal is fairly new, but the content is expanding every day. The website has a link to listings of prolotherapy physicians, as well as information about prolotherapy research.

You can also ask your doctor, chiropractor, physical therapist, or other health care provider for a reference.

Appendix B

Why News of Prolotherapy Hasn't Spread

One of the questions I hear more than almost any other, after "What is prolotherapy," is "Why haven't I heard of prolotherapy?" The answer speaks to some of the problems with the American health care system. When the injury is a broken bone, there is probably no better treatment than that given by an orthopedist trained in the United States. Deformities of any kind receive incredible, innovative treatments from our plastic surgeons. But when the injury is less obvious, as with soft tissue injuries, the American health care system fails us.

In 1991, I was doing my second residency in occupational and preventive medicine at the University of Arizona. During that time, I saw the difficulty in treating common occupational injuries, such as soft tissue injuries in the back, and the limits of orthopedic surgery in being able to successfully return people to work. Here I was first exposed to chiropractic medicine and the treatment of soft tissue injuries. Many patients recovered from seemingly intractable pain with manual medicine techniques. The improvements were not miraculous or instantaneous, but took considerable time and patience. The chiropractors always seemed to get the people whose pain generator was somewhat unidentifiable. But they were successful in helping many of these people return to active, healthy lives.

However, the idea that "to cut is to cure," as the surgeons would often tell me, is very deeply ingrained in U.S. medicine. Yes, there is a very significant difference in the level of education and training for chiropractors and orthopedists. But sometimes the ego of a physician gets in the way of his or her clinical judgment.

As physicians we very much want to heal the patient who comes to us in pain. And during my time at the University of Arizona, it became obvious to me that surgery was a bit of a crapshoot, with many patients obtaining incredible relief, while others remained the same or became much worse. And there was a huge jump in the risks of the treatments given by a primary care physician or chiropractor and a surgeon. In the patients we saw, if the pain wasn't too bad, they could live with it, taking analgesics or narcotics as needed. But if the pain was too severe, prevented them from working, or impeded an active lifestyle, having exhausted all other options, they would take a chance on surgery.

When I questioned what other treatment could be given for those in constant, sometimes severe pain who refused to receive surgery, a naturopathic doctor suggested I read the book *Pain, Pain, Go Away* by William Faber and Morton Walker, doctor of osteopathic medicine. I read it with great interest. It was written for the lay public, and it was not a scientific medical book. However, it made a lot of sense. The explanation given for the cause of many instances of chronic pain could help bridge the gap between simple treatment failures and surgery. And prolotherapy could help separate, in my opinion, patients who would do well with surgery from those who may not be helped by surgery.

But then I thought, "This can't be." If prolotherapy was half as successful as these authors described, I would have heard of it. In five years of residency training, first as a family physician and later as an occupational and preventive physician rotating through orthopedic and sports medicine, never had I heard of prolotherapy. Faber must be a quack, I thought. The fact that he was charging several thousand dollars to train others in the technique made me only more suspicious. Particularly considering that I was a low-paid resident, I had a lot of school debt to pay, and my first child had just been born. Taking a chance by traveling to the Milwaukee Pain Clinic was too daunting, and I didn't give the subject much further thought.

At that same time another physician I knew was practicing psychiatry. The practice of psychiatry was not what he had hoped for, and he was looking to do something else. He had also read Dr. Faber's book, but he was not as cynical. He was single, and he had the money available to take a chance. What he learned began to change the lives of many patients. With my doubts erased, I had him teach me the treatment. I received further training from the American Academy of Orthopaedic Medicine (AAOM). Since that time, I know I have made a very positive change in hundreds of lives. If I had not learned of prolotherapy, I only wonder how many of those individuals would continue to be in pain and unable to work or live happy, active lives.

By 1992, I had gone into private practice as a family practitioner in Pasadena, Texas, close to where I was born and raised in Houston, Texas. I was full of enthusiasm and idealism. Finally, I was ready to try to improve people's lives by improving their health. I did not plan on just treating the symptoms of chronic diseases such as high blood pressure, diabetes, heart disease, and the like. Through my training as a preventive medicine physician, I was going to address the underlying conditions, such as obesity, diet, stress, and lack of exercise. Hopefully, I would be able to eliminate the diseases by addressing lifestyle changes. I planned to teach patients to eliminate the need for medication by changing bad habits. Prolotherapy fit perfectly into my philosophy because it treated the underlying causes of chronic pain— weakened ligaments and tendons.

I enrolled in courses sponsored by the AAOM, and learned more about the science behind prolotherapy and was instructed on its application. The academy is composed of many dedicated physicians who are intent on making the benefits of prolotherapy better known and who are generous in sharing their vast experience. This to me was medicine at its best. Many highly trained physicians in prolotherapy were giving of their knowledge and experience without regard for compensation. The many physicians in the AAOM worked hard to promote prolotherapy, not to become rich, but because they felt it was the right thing to do.

Returning to my practice, I began to apply prolotherapy to the many patients who would come to me complaining of musculoskeletal pain. When simple analgesics, rest, and physical therapy did not relieve the pain, I offered them prolotherapy. Initially, I was amazed to see most of these people get well. Some, of course, did not improve and were referred on to orthopedists for further evaluation and treatment.

After attending a marketing course for physicians and dentists, I decided to advertise. They recommended using testimonials as a way to attract patients. An advertisement placed in a Houston newspaper was quite successful. Patients sometimes came from over a hundred miles away. For the first time, I began treating patients whose pain was chronic, lasting sometimes many years. Even in those cases I would see significant success. Relieving someone of his or her chronic pain was very satisfying.

Through word of mouth, patients whom orthopedists were unable to help or who wanted a treatment that did not involve surgery were coming to see me. Many of these patients also did well. Soon I realized I had something special on my hands. I wasn't sure why it wasn't more commonly used, but now I had proof that it worked.

Shortly thereafter, I received a notice that changed everything. The Texas Medical Board was initiating an investigation into my ads. Someone had called to complain that I had used a testimonial in my ad. A recent change in the rules had made it illegal for physicians to use testimonials in their ads. The Medical Board felt it was inappropriate for physicians to use examples of treatment successes because patients may be duped into thinking they too could achieve the same exact benefit from the same treatment. I asked physicians in my community about the rule change and the vast majority were also unaware of it. It seemed unlikely to me that an ordinary citizen made the complaint, and I didn't think I had any patients who were dissatisfied with their treatment. I thought the complaint had to have been made by a knowledgeable physician. My ads contained real patients with their actual statements about how prolotherapy had helped them.

When I learned of the rule change, I changed my ads immediately. Yet at the time, there were many cases of testimonials being used by physicians, particularly plastic surgeons. Their ads typically contained before and after pictures, thus implying that you could get the same results. They were not investigated. "Why not just tell me to change my ad," I thought. But for reasons not clear to me my ad garnered special attention.

I was asked to gather all of the records of the patients I had treated with prolotherapy and send copies of them to the Medical Board. This was no simple task for a physician just starting out in practice. But I had to comply. I felt that once they discovered that it was simply a mistake and that I had immediately changed the ad, they would go back to spending their time investigating dangerous and unethical physicians. At the time, the Texas Medical Board was being criticized for being too lax in their investigation and enforcement of these practices. I was wrong. A date was set for me to go before the Board.

A civilian representative, a physician appointed by the governor, and a representative from the attorney general's office were waiting for me. To my surprise, for about an hour all the questions were related to prolotherapy. Where was I trained, how many did I do, how much did I charge, where did the patients come from and so on. The civilian did all the talking, at least in terms of criticizing prolotherapy. When I mentioned that the former surgeon general of the United States endorsed the use of prolotherapy, he said C. Everett Koop had been misled. I wondered why this nonphysician had suddenly become more knowledgeable about medicine than our former surgeon general and was telling me that my experience with prolotherapy was wrong. The physician present was curiously silent. The last five minutes of the inquiry were spent on the specifics of the ad.

I was told that if I would forego a formal trial and pay a two thousand dollar administrative fine nothing would go on my permanent record. At that point, I was willing to get it behind me for two thousand dollars. Unfortunately, I was deceived. A report was sent to the Medical Board Clearing House, making my life with insurance companies miserable for several months while I explained the charge.

Licensing boards are appointed by the state to help ensure the competency of the physicians allowed to practice in that state. In Texas, the requirements are successfully finishing a medical degree program at an accredited medical school, passing the required exams, and completing at least one year of an approved medical internship. Naturally physicians make up a significant part of any medical board because they have the knowledge necessary to judge competency. However, in the case of the prolotherapy ad, competency was not the issue and similar ads were not similarly dealt with. Board members are part-time officials and the appointments are political. They may have a direct economic interest in the decisions they make. Some members may even represent certain specialties within the medical profession. After my experience with the Board, I was left with the feeling that their action against me had less to do with protecting the public and more to do with limiting the practice and knowledge of prolotherapy, and thus limiting competition within the profession.

Prolotherapy Isn't Patentable

My experience left me with the realization that prolotherapy was different from other nontraditional treatments. The fact that prolotherapy uses very simple substances to provoke a healing response is one of its greatest strengths and one of its greatest weaknesses. It is impossible to obtain a patent on a simple substance such as glucose. Who then was going to spend the exorbitant amounts of money for large, in-depth studies? Who was going to invest large sums of money to educate and promote the use of prolotherapy among physicians?

We need look no further than the debacle of Premarin and Provera to see how pharmaceutical companies and their desire to find patentable drugs to market can harm the American health care consumer. As our hormones drop with age, maintaining a certain low level of estrogen and progesterone in women is beneficial in many ways, including the maintenance of bone strength, improved cardiovascular disease risk, and improved mood. Logically, one would replace the depleted hormones with substances having an identical chemical structure. However, this is not what was done because naturally occurring human estrogen and progesterone cannot be patented. Instead, a pharmaceutical company spent large sums of money convincing doctors with their studies that Premarin and Provera were the ideal hormonal replacement therapy for women. Premarin is an estrogen natural to a horse and obtained from pregnant mares' urine—not even the same species. Provera is even worse. It is artificially made progesterone not natural to any animal. Eventually, it was shown that these two drugs might induce cancer. Because of this and the fear of lawsuits, physicians stopped prescribing hormonal replacement to any woman, despite the known benefits and the strong desire of women to take it due to the significant improvement in their sense of well-being. (*Note:* An excellent book for anyone considering hormonal replacement, including men, is *Hormones, Health, and Happiness* (2007) by Dr. Steven F. Hotze. Bioidentical hormones are easily available at compounding pharmacies with significant benefit both physically and mentally. The ability of companies to increase profits with patentable medications can distort the recommendations a physician makes about many medical conditions. Treatments that cannot be patented, such as prolotherapy, are ignored—or worse—to the great detriment of many people.

Several years ago, a friend and colleague with whom I attended the preventive medicine program at the University of Arizona called me. During our conversation, he mentioned he was writing a book. It was to describe the benefits of a simple substance in the treatment of arthritis. The medication was a simple supplement you could obtain from a health food store. I didn't think it would go anywhere. I was wrong. It made the *New York Times* bestseller list. The supplement, glucosamine, can now be found at any pharmacy thanks to the book *Arthritis Cure* by Jason Theodosakis. In many ways, this supplement is better than the expensive pharmaceutical drugs commonly prescribed. I recommend glucosamine to all of my patients receiving prolotherapy. Despite the fact that many of my patients responded very well to glucosamine, the orthopedic surgeons were originally derisive of the supplement, telling my patients it was a waste of money. After being proven wrong, they have been willing to accept it. Unfortunately, it is not always an arthritis cure but it does help. For some it helps a lot. Glucosamine would never have seen the light of day had it not been for the book. Again, no patent, no support.

Prolotherapy Isn't a Moneymaker

The fact that prolotherapy uses substances too simple to patent is a serious mark against it. That alone would make it worthy of being ignored, but something else makes many in the medical community hostile toward it. Sometimes, even in the practice of medicine, it's all about money.

Recently, I was involved in helping our community get a new hospital. The Pasadena area had four hospitals when I started practicing but had dropped to one within a decade. Many physicians felt the quality of health care provided by the remaining hospital was suffering. We decided to inject some good old American competition by starting a hospital. In doing the due diligence required to determine the likelihood of success for this hospital, we learned that a large portion of the revenue and profits come from orthopedic surgeries. Hospitals are already struggling with the expense of caring for the uninsured; so to offer a treatment that could significantly decrease the need for orthopedic surgeries, like prolotherapy, would no doubt hurt financially and not be welcomed.

For the orthopedic surgeons who have endured the long road through medical school and residency training with long hours and low pay, to finish is finally payday. They deserve to be paid very well for all the knowledge, training, and expense they have had to endure. Their ability to repair our broken and shattered bones is incredible. But to be paid well one must do surgeries — and preferably often. So when they hear that a well-trained family practitioner can reduce the need for surgery with prolotherapy, they aren't likely very happy or positive about the treatment.

I have had hundreds of patients cancel their surgeries or refuse surgery after successfully completing prolotherapy. I understand the hostility toward prolotherapy and the desire to discredit the procedure, but in the end we must do what is in the best interest of the patient. We still must be guided by the maxim "Do no harm."

An extreme case of greed and incompetence can be found in Eric Heston Scheffey, referred to in a *Texas Monthly* article in September 2005 as Dr. Evil ("Dr. Evil" by S.C. Gwynne). Despite overwhelming evidence of his incompetence (at the time of the article, he had been sued seventy-eight times for malpractice), he was able to both keep his license and continue operating. Several people died and many were maimed from his surgeries, most of which were deemed unnecessary. They were deemed unnecessary only in hindsight. In the Texas Workers' Compensation system, all surgeries have to be reviewed by another surgeon to certify that the surgery is necessary. As one of the leading billers of the workers' compensation system, he was always able to find another physician to agree to the need for surgery, even when it was the second or third operation on the same patient. Despite losing his privileges at several hospitals, he was able to find a place to operate. Surgicenters in search of profits, as well as small hospitals, allowed Dr. Scheffey to operate; he quickly became their main revenue producer. There are other physicians like Dr. Scheffey. Unfortunately, there will always be a small percentage of physicians and health care facilities that do not operate with the patient's best interest in mind.

I have cared for some of Dr. Scheffey's patients. They will never have normal lives. They will be in constant pain and will need serious drugs for the rest of their lives.

Misleading Prolotherapy Studies

Prolotherapy is allowed in the Texas Workers' Compensation system, but many times it is deemed medically unnecessary. Because of abuses that have occurred in the system resulting in huge costs to the employers of the state, now even surgeries that are necessary are delayed or denied as medically unnecessary. It is the insurance companies that are now abusing the employees.

One of the greatest criticisms against prolotherapy is its lack of double-blind studies. Good studies have been done, but for some critics there are never enough. The studies that have not supported prolotherapy have been poorly constructed, but many people don't understand that. Recently, I was speaking to a physician during a peer-to-peer review of a request to do prolotherapy on a patient who had hurt his lower back. Peer-to-peer reviews are necessary for insurance companies and are conducted by physicians who are hired by the insurance company to help them determine the appropriateness of treatment plans for injured workers. This is a perfectly reasonable thing to do to prevent excessive and uncoordinated care. As soon as I got on the phone, the physician began to quote the fact that the Workers' Compensation Guidelines state that prolotherapy is experimental. When I asked her if she knew anything about prolotherapy, she immediately responded that she had researched the treatment and found it to have no merit. How did she come to that conclusion, I asked.

Again, she was quick to refer to an article on a randomized trial by M.J. Yelland and colleagues as proof of prolotherapy's lack of worth as a treatment. The article published in the January 2004 edition of *Spine*, was titled "Prolotherapy Injections, Saline Injections, and Exercises for Chronic Low-back Pain: A Randomized Study," and it concluded that prolotherapy is no better than a placebo treatment. Unfortunately, the author did not understand prolotherapy very well and made some mistakes, as I explained to the insurance company physician. Dr. Yelland used a 20 percent glucose solution as his prolotherapy solution and normal saline as his placebo. What Dr. Yelland did not realize is that normal saline is used in prolotherapy and is considered a weak proliferant solution. Even dry needling without any solution can promote inflammation and therefore healing (see chapter 7).

What the insurance physician failed to realize is that the study showed that both solutions when injected into the ligaments of patients with chronic nonspecific low back pain had significant and sustained reductions in pain and disability. The study should have tested prolotherapy against an actual placebo or nontreatment. Instead it was a strong prolotherapy solution versus a weak prolotherapy solution. Although the stronger solution did better in reducing pain and disability, the difference was not statistically significant. You would think that the study conclusion demonstrating an improvement in the pain and disability of chronic low back pain with a simple injection into the ligaments would result in further studies to find out why. Instead it was being used as a reason to deny a patient the opportunity to receive prolotherapy. Pointing out these facts to the insurance physician did not appear to sway her opinion of prolotherapy. Unfortunately, her mind was made up before she got on the phone.

In the past, many great discoveries were made through thoughtful experience. Doctors would see patterns and discover new illnesses. Treatments were sometimes discovered by accident or through trial and error. Cures were studied and repeated and if a benefit was noted, that treatment would become part of a physician's regimen for that disease. Penicillin was used for many years before we knew exactly how it worked. You would think that clinical data showing prolotherapy has cured thousands of patients over the years would lead to serious research and its greater use in the health care system.

Medical devices, however, do not seem to get the same scrutiny for some reason. Despite, or perhaps because of, the estimated $80 billion a year spent on medical devices the industry was barely regulated until 1976, when the FDA began to evaluate devices for safety, effectiveness, and quality. An exception to the law passed by Congress states that a medical device can be accepted with little or no clinical trials if it is concluded to be "substantially equivalent" to a medical device that existed prior to 1976.

Johnson and Johnson has a metal device, known as the Charité, for chronic back pain due to an injured disc. This has now been implanted into thousands of spines in patients whose back pain did not respond to the usual remedies. The FDA approved this after a trial of only 304 patients. Of those patients, only 36 percent improved enough to suspend their narcotic analgesics. In an article published in *Forbes* magazine on November 27, 2006, ("Dangerous Devices," Matthew Herper and Robert Langreth) Catherine Rich, 40, speaks of experiencing significant back pain for only three months before being convinced to have this $11,500 device inserted into her spine. She is quoted as saying, "It was presented like it was going to solve all my problems." Her back pain unfortunately returned more severe than ever. Another surgery later, her back pain was still severe, requiring her to spend nearly all of her day in a special bed. She felt the surgeries ruined her life. Some estimate that hundreds of other patients have been made worse through the use of Charité and at least 30 of those patients have now sued Johnson and Johnson. At the same time many patients are cured of seemingly intractable pain. So which is it? Is the Charité a valuable implant or is it worthless. The answer is, it depends. If the pain is the result of the disc it may very well result in an improvement in the patient's pain level, but if the cause is a soft tissue injury the surgery can only make it worse. Unfortunately, choice of patients is probably at fault. The trouble is, if surgeons only choose those patients most likely to benefit from the prosthesis using more rigorous criteria, then they may not be able to perform as many surgeries. Physicians have a very difficult time separating those whose pain is originating from a disc injury from other patients with back pain. And it's very difficult to separate those whose back pain is a result of a soft tissue injury if you don't want to know about or are uninformed about soft tissue injuries.

Competition — Putting Treatment Decisions into the Hands of the Patient

The fall of Soviet Union settled once and for all the question of whether centrally-planned economies are inferior to market-based economies. There is no way a committee of intelligent people can compete with the innovation, ideas, and energy of millions of free men and women. And yet the United States, the greatest bastion of free enterprise, fails to utilize its own system of capitalism in health care. We have our health insurance companies micromanaging treatments, providers, and prices. Entrusting our insurance companies and government to manage our health care system has resulted in millions of Americans without health care, expenses that have been outpacing inflation, and incredible inequality.

In the marketplace, ideas are constantly being tested. A new technology that completely changes the way a job or activity is done is referred to as a disruptive technology. Disruptive technologies that improve efficiency to the benefit of society are soon adopted. You can bet the makers of typewriters would have loved to have prevented the introduction of the word processor. Or what about the introduction of digital photography. How many people still put Kodak film in their cameras? Would any society give Kodak, because of their expertise, the exclusive right to determine what cameras or films could be sold in the United States?

Unfortunately, this does happen in health care.

Why prolotherapy is not more commonly utilized to heal injuries without resorting to costly and sometimes inappropriate surgery speaks to the lack of competition in the health care system. It wasn't until years after I started using it that I realized what a disruptive technology prolotherapy is. If prolotherapy were to become a more commonplace alterative to surgery, billions of dollars could be saved through the elimination of unnecessary surgeries, hospitalizations, anesthesiology, complications, rehabilitation, and disability. Therein lies the problem. If society saves billions of dollars through the elimination of unnecessary surgeries, then it is the doctors and facilities that lose the billions of dollars.

Most people believe that even if physicians are not actively working to limit health care costs, surely the insurance companies are working hard to control them. But insurance companies are merely middlemen between the patients' money and the providers of care. They add up the bills and demand a premium to cover their costs. The insurance companies rely on physicians to help them determine the standard of care. But there is little scrutiny of those who develop the standards of care.

Although there are good reasons for developing standards of treatment, they are also very anticompetitive. Many innovative treatments are excluded by accident or design. It's not fair to expect insurance companies to evaluate all the possible medical treatments that exist, so the physicians they turn to must be open to all of the possible treatments that are available and that have been shown to work time and time again.

Medicine has the danger of group think, often following recommendations from experts who were very narrowly trained and who therefore have a very limited perspective on the best treatment options.

Insurance companies have failed to ask why there are so many cases of failed back syndrome. Even given the many cases showing total resolution of injuries through the use of prolotherapy, there is an unwillingness to consider another option in the back pain algorithm. The lack of an open mind can lead to disastrous results.

The marketplace may already be addressing the lack of competition in the health care arena. More and more companies and individuals have turned to high-deductible major medical plans as well as health care savings accounts (HSA). As more patients turn to alternative medicine for their health care needs, they increasingly see insurance companies as too restrictive in their coverage of benefits. Prolotherapy, as an example, is practiced by hundreds of board certified physicians across the country that regularly do research and education through the AAOM, but it is frequently not a covered benefit. People are increasingly rejecting insurance companies that pay for expensive procedures but won't cover inexpensive alternatives. They are extremely frustrated to have paid premiums for years only to find that the insurance company will not pay for the treatment they feel is most appropriate for them and their conditions. With patients able to choose their care more freely and having to pay out of their own pockets, a level of competition will emerge not seen since the advent of employer-based health insurance.

Appendix C

Letter from C. Everett Koop

 DEPARTMENT OF HEALTH & HUMAN SERVICES

The Surgeon General of the
Public Health Service
Rockville MD 20857

AUG 2 2 1986

Everett Nicholas, M.D.
1 Erie Court
Oak Park, Illinois 60302

Dear Dr. Nicholas:

This is in response to your request for a statement concerning prolotherapy. I respond as a patient who has benefited from it and as a
practicing surgeon who used it successfully, but certainly not in my
official capacity as the Surgeon General of the U.S. Public Health
Service.

I think that prolotherapy is an effective method of pain relief, when
properly practiced. Prolotherapy frequently works when all other therapy
has failed. I say this in spite of the fact that official groups and some
insurance companies have taken a contrary point of view. I cannot help but
believe these decisions are made in ignorance or because of conflicts of
interest.

I was diagnosed as having intractable pain by two neurologic groups in
prominent academic institutions, but was totally relieved of my symptoms
when treated by Dr. Hemwall at West Suburban Hospital in Illinois. I have
benefited from this therapy on a number of occasions since that time.

As a surgeon I found very little use for prolotherapy in my practice, which
was confined to children. However, on many occasions I was able to relieve
my patients' parents of pain by using the techniques I had learned from
Dr. Hemwall.

I trust this information will be helpful to you.

Sincerely yours,

C. Everett Koop, M.D.
Surgeon General

Glossary

acupressure — Therapy that applies pressure, as with thumbs and fingertips, to points on the body to relieve tension or pain

acute pain — Pain associated with small injuries (that don't last long or cause permanent damage) because of the inflammatory process that occurs; generally somatic pain

analgesic — Any drug or medication that is used to relieve pain

annulus fibrosus — See fibrocartilage

anterior cruciate ligament (ACL) — Ligament that extends from upper back to lower front of the knee, connecting the tibia and the femur

anterolisthesis — Movement of the vertebral bodies forward, out of normal alignment

arachnoiditis — Inflammatory condition that may follow trauma, tumor, infections, bleeding, or administration of various compounds into the spinal fluid; can cause neck and back pain

arthritis — Breakdown of cartilage as a result of wear and tear, injury, obesity, and broken bones; symptoms include morning stiffness, pain upon movement, cracking, swelling, and redness of joints, and loss of flexibility

arthroplasty — Joint replacement surgery (most often for the knees and hips) in cases of severe deterioration of the components of a joint from osteoarthritis or some other degenerative condition; the procedure uses an artificial joint made of metal and plastic

articular — Of or relating to a joint

articular cartilage — Material that makes up the opposing side of the bones that form synovial joints; it does not contain any blood vessels or nerves

avascular — Lacking blood vessels

back extension — Skeletal irregularity in which the spine bends backward

back flexion — Skeletal irregularity in which the spine bends forward

botulinum toxin — Neurotoxin protein produced by the bacterium Clostridium botulinum; used in minute doses to treat painful muscle spasms, though it is very toxic in high doses

bulging disc — Condition where the annulus fibrosus becomes weak in a certain spot and bulges outward

bursas — Small, fluid-filled sacs between a tendon and a bone that provide cushioning and reduce friction

bursitis — Inflammation in a joint (commonly shoulders and elbows) of the bursas

C nerve fibers — Pain-specific nerve terminals within the substance of normal intervertebral discs themselves; proliferate abnormally in degenerated discs, potentially making them more prone to pain than normal discs

carpal tunnel syndrome — Compression of the median nerve that runs from the forearm into the hand by the carpal tunnel (a rigid passage of ligament and bones at the base of the hand); common symptom is numbness or tingling in the palm of the hand near the wrist or thumb

cartilage — Translucent, somewhat elastic tissue composed of water (65–80 percent), collagen, and proteoglycans (the latter components are produced by chondrocytes)

cervical spine — Neck area of the spinal column; has seven vertebrae

chiropractic — Therapy that uses manipulation and specific adjustment of such body structures as the spine to treat pain

chondrocytes — Specialized cells that perform specific functions throughout the body; they exist within synovial tissue

chronic pain — Pain that lasts longer than three to six months or beyond the point when tissue has healed; can be either somatic or neuropathic

collagen — Any of a group of fibrous proteins that are the main substance in connective tissues and bones

computerized tomography (CT) — See CT scan

connective tissue — Soft tissue, usually in our tendons, ligaments, and muscles, that is prone to injury

corticosteroids — See steroids

costovertebral junctions — Points at which the ribs are joined to the vertebral bodies

CT scan — Computerized tomography scan; a medical imaging method where digital geometry processing is used to generate a three-dimensional image of the inside of an object from a large series of two-dimensional X-ray images taken around a single axis of rotation

dermatomal pain — Referred nerve pain patterns

diffusion — Process by which cartilage is able to absorb nutrients because they naturally pass from a fluid where they are highly concentrated to the cells in the cartilage where they are less concentrated

discectomy — Surgical procedure to remove a spinal disc; typically done when a disc has herniated or ruptured and the goal is to remove the tissue that is putting pressure on the spinal cord or the nerve roots, and causing pain

discogenic pain — Pain that comes from inside the disc itself as a result of its degeneration

dynamic radiographic computerized analysis — Method that involves taking a series of X-rays while the body/body part is in different positions (flexion, extension, and neutral) and marking specific points on the vertebral bodies in the images to demonstrate ligament laxity

electro muscle stimulation (EMS) — Technique to trigger muscle contraction to calm muscle spasms, rehabilitate and reeducate atrophied muscles, increase or restore range of motion, and facilitate recovery from surgery or medical therapy

electromyography — Nerve and muscle study

facet arthritis — Debilitating pain as a result of facet joint deterioration; also known as degenerative joint disease of the spine, facet arthropathy, or spondylosis

facet denervation — Radiofrequency ablation used in the facet joints of the spine

facet joints — Small joints that occur on each side of the vertebrae in the spine to connect them; the only joints that do not contain synovial fluid

failed back syndrome — Chronic back and/or leg pain that occurs after back or spinal surgery; also known as failed back surgery

fibrocartilage — Tough, flexible, and elastic substance on outside of each disc that is a combination of cartilage and fibrous connective tissue; also known as the annulus fibrosus

foraminotomy — Surgical procedure to remove bone from around the neuroforamen to widen the passage and relieve pressure on the nerve roots

glucocorticoids — See steroids

golfer's elbow (medial epicondylitis) — Similar to tennis elbow, but it affects the inside of the elbow

herniated disc — Condition where a weakened point in a bulging disc ruptures, releasing the nucleus pulposus it contains

hyaline cartilage — Cartilage that makes up the ends of the articulating (opposing) bones in synovial joints; also known as articular cartilage

hypermobility — Joints that stretch farther than is normal; also known as "double-jointed"

iliolumbar ligament — Ligament that connects the lower spine to the pelvis

ilium — Broad, dorsal, upper, and largest of the three bones that compose either half of the pelvis

inflammation — Reaction of the body to injury or to infectious, allergic, or chemical irritation; symptoms are redness, swelling, heat, and pain resulting from dilation of the blood vessels in the affected part with loss of plasma and leucocytes into the tissues

intervertebral discs — Tiny little round gel packs that lie between adjacent vertebrae and, together with the vertebrae on either side of them, form a joint; act as pillows to absorb or distribute forces applied to the spine

intradiscal electrothermoplasty — Procedure in which a wire is temporarily inserted into a disc and heated to destroy the sensory nerves; cannot be conducted on severely degenerated discs

joint capsule — Space between bones because they are not directly connected; also known as chamber

kyphosis — Skeletal irregularity in which the normal curve of the upper back is severely rounded

laminectomy — Removal of lamina (the bony plate at the back of each vertebra that protects the spinal column) or a vertebra or a section of vertebrae; usually performed to correct a condition called spinal stenosis

lateral collateral ligament (LCL) — Ligament that runs along the outside of the knee

lateral epicondylitis — See tennis elbow

leucocytes/lymphocytes — White blood cells

leukotrienes — Act as transporters of the necessary cells to the injured tissues in the healing process, controlling whether the blood vessels allow those cells to pass through the vessel walls and come in contact with the injured tissues

ligament laxity — Loose ligaments

ligaments — Tough, dense strands of connective tissue (composed of collagen fiber) that join bones to other bones or to cartilage in the joint areas; form the joint capsule and hold every synovial joint together

lordosis — Skeletal irregularity in which there's an abnormally accentuated arch in the lower back

lumbar spine — Lower back area of spinal column; has five vertebrae

medial collateral ligament (MCL) — Ligament that runs along the inside of knee

medial epicondylitis — See golfer's elbow

meniscus — Fibrous cartilage within a joint, especially of the knee

minimally invasive surgery — Term that refers to surgery performed using laparoscopic or endoscopic methods; typically requires two or more very small incisions

MRI — Magnetic resonance imaging; a medical imaging technique commonly used in radiology to visualize the structure and function of the body; provides much greater contrast between the different soft tissues of the body than computerized tomography does

myelograms — Contrast X-rays using an injected dye into the spinal cavity to highlight the space between the bony structures, offering a better view of the spinal cord and nerve roots

myofascial pain syndrome — Chronic muscle pain

myofascial release — Soft tissue therapy, similar to massage, to loosen the fibers of various fascia components by stretching them and breaking bonds that have formed between connective tissues and other soft tissues through scarring, improper healing of injuries, or repeated misuse of those tissues

neuroforamen — Passageways between the vertebrae that exist on either side of the spine; nerve roots that extend from the spinal cord run through these passageways

neuro-muscular electro stimulation (NMES) — Like EMS, a technique to trigger muscle contraction to calm muscle spasms, rehabilitate and reeducate atrophied muscles, increase or restore range of motion, and facilitate recovery from surgery or medical therapy

neuropathic pain — Nerve pain caused by amputation, chemotherapy, diabetes, HIV infection, multiple sclerosis, shingles, or surgery, particularly spinal surgery; manifests as burning or tingling or numbness

nociceptors — Sensory receptors in the form of nerve endings

nonpharmacological — Not related to therapeutic drugs

NSAIDs — Non-steroidal anti-inflammatory drugs; they have analgesic, antipyretic, and, in higher doses, anti-inflammatory effects such as reducing pain, fever, and inflammation

nucleus pulposus — Inner core of each intervertebral disc

open surgery — Term that refers to surgery that requires opening a cavity in the body in order to perform the surgery; typically involves making larger incisions and cutting through fascia, muscle, and possibly other soft tissues

osteoarthritis — Clinical syndrome in which low-grade inflammation results in pain in the joints; caused by abnormal wearing of the cartilage that covers and acts as a cushion inside joints and destruction or decrease of synovial fluid that lubricates those joints

osteonecrosis — Condition that occurs when blood flow to the bone is restricted

osteophyte — Bony outgrowth from the vertebral body, possibly resulting from an old calcified injury

osteoporosis — Condition marked by a decreased amount of bone

osteoporotic vertebral fractures — Bone fractures (particularly in lower back) that can occur from a fall or even from the stress of lifting or everyday activities due to osteoporosis

pain centralization — Process whereby certain nerve cells in the brain and spinal cord (the central nervous system) are abnormally activated and maintain and even augment the sensation of pain

pelvic spine — Tailbone area of the spinal column; has several fused sacral and coccygeal vertebrae

PENS — Percutaneous electrical nerve stimulation system

"phantom limb syndrome" — When patient experiences pain in a previously amputated limb because certain brain circuitries abnormally maintain or even increase the level of perceived pain in an arm or a leg that is no longer there

plantar fasciitis — Painful inflammatory condition of the foot caused by excessive pressure to the arch of the foot

platelet-rich plasma (PRP) — Blood derivative with a more concentrated level of platelets than ordinary blood and tissue growth factors that can help heal ligaments and tendons; also known as autologous platelet concentrate, platelet leukocyte gel, platelet-rich plasma gel, platelet concentrate, and blood plasma therapy

posterior cruciate ligament (PCL) — Ligament that extends from the upper front to the lower back of the knee joint, also connecting to the tibia and the femur

prolotherapist — Physician trained to do prolotherapy

prolotherapy — Treatment in the region of tendons or ligaments for the purpose of strengthening weakened connective tissue and alleviating musculoskeletal pain; involves injecting a non-pharmacological solution (often dextrose, a sugar solution) that restores cartilage and strengthens ligaments and tendons; also known as proliferative therapy, reconstructive therapy, or a type of regenerative injection therapy

prostoglandin — Biochemical found in nearly all of the body's tissues and organs

proteoglycans — Any of a class of glycoproteins of high molecular weight found especially in the extracellular matrix of connective tissue

radiofrequency ablation — Technique developed to accurately and effectively treat a small volume of sensory nerve tissue, thereby disrupting transmission of pain signals along a specific nerve

referred pain — Condition where pain is actually referred to (or hurts at) a site on the body other than where the injury originates; occurs with many soft tissue injuries

repetitive strain injury (RSI) — Condition that results from repetitive use of a limb, particularly the arms; symptoms include pain that worsens with activity, inflammation, stiffness, weakness or lack of endurance, and nerve pain; also known as repetitive stress injury

retrolisthesis — Movement of the vertebral bodies backward, out of normal alignment

rheumatoid arthritis — Chronic and progressively degenerative and inflammatory condition in which the immune system attacks its own joints and tissues in the skin, blood vessels, heart, lungs, and muscles

sacroiliac — Juncture of the sacrum and the ilium

sacroiliac (SI) joint—Joint between the base of the spine, the sacrum, and the iliac crest of the pelvis

sacrotuberous ligament—Ligament situated in the lower back part of the pelvis that connects the sacrum to the lower part of the hipbone

sacrum—Base of the spine

scleratomal pain patterns—Referred pain patterns caused by soft tissue injuries

scoliosis—Skeletal irregularity in which the spine curves to the side

soft tissue—Tissues that connect, support, or surround other structures and organs of the body; includes muscles, tendons, ligaments, fascia, fibrous tissues, fat, blood vessels, and synovial membranes

soft tissue injury—Type of injury most commonly involving tendons, ligaments, and muscles—sometimes all three

somatic pain—Pain that results from sensory receptors in the form of nerve endings actually reacting to the mechanical, thermal, or chemical changes that are occurring in damaged tissues (ligaments, tendons, muscle, bones, and fascia)

spinal fusion—Procedure that involves a bone graft to the front, back, or side of a vertebral pair (or even multiple vertebrae) to fill an area where bone from the vertebrae or the disc is missing; treatment for spondylolisthesis and scoliosis

spinal stenosis—Condition where the canals in your vertebra that allow the spinal cord to run through the spine or that allow the nerve roots to exit the spinal column narrow

spondylolisthesis—Condition where there is an abnormal displacement of one vertebra over another, which causes damage to the spinal nerves. Anterior displacement of a vertebra or the vertebral column in relation to the vertebrae below

spondylolysis—Defect in the pars interarticularis of a vertebra; typically caused by stress fracture of the bone and is associated with certain activities, such as dance, weight lifting, and gymnastics

sprain—Stretching or wrenching of the ligaments and tendons of a joint, often with rupture of the tissues but without dislocation; symptoms include inflammation, pain, swelling, and loss of function

steroids (corticosteroids or glucocorticoids)—Synthetic forms of cortisol, which is naturally produced by the adrenal system in the body to regulate inflammation

strain—Injury to a muscle in which the muscle fibers tear as a result of overstretching

subluxation—Incomplete or partial dislocation of a joint or an organ; in chiropractic and other manual medicines, refers to the improper alignment or juxtaposition of vertebrae with the surrounding vertebrae

synovial fluid—Fluid that carries nutrients to cartilage; it is created by the synovial membrane, or synovium

synovial joints—Joints that offer the most range of movement and, consequently, are the least stable and the most prone to injury; formed where two or more bones meet but are not directly joined to each other; include the shoulder, elbow, wrist, hip, knee, and ankle joints

synovial tissue—Tissue that is found between the articular cartilages and contained by the joint capsule

synovitis—Inflammation of the synovium, particularly the synovial lining, as a result of inflammatory or even noninflammatory joint diseases; symptoms include swelling in and around the joint that is visible to the naked eye

synovium—Thin lining of the joint capsule, or chamber; also a protective sheath covering tendons to protect them from friction as other structures move over them; also known as the synovial membrane

Synvisc—Product containing hyaluronic acid (the major component of synovial fluid) that improves effectiveness of prolotherapy (for osteoarthritis in the knees especially) by increasing the fluid in our joints and thereby the cushioning and lubrication of the joint

tendinitis—Irritation and inflammation of a tendon (commonly in shoulders, elbows, wrists, and heels) as a result of overuse; symptoms include pain (near related joint), tenderness, and mild swelling

tendinosis—Damage to a tendon at a cellular level, causing fibers of the tendon to fray or deteriorate; symptoms include pain upon use, tenderness, swelling, and inflammation

tendon—Tough cord composed of closely packed white fibers of connective tissue that serves to attach muscles to internal structures such as bones or other muscles

tennis elbow (lateral epicondylitis)—Inflammation and possible degeneration of the tendon in the forearm that connects to the lateral epicondyle (bulge at the end of the upper arm bone); symptoms include pain radiating from the outside of the elbow, down the forearm, to the back of the hand

tenosynovitis—Inflammation of the sheath that surrounds a tendon (commonly wrists, hands, and feet) as a result of injury, strain, overuse, or infection; symptoms include pain, stiffness, inflammation, and swelling of a joint

TENS system—Transcutaneous electrical nerve stimulation

thoracic spine—Chest area of the spinal column; has twelve vertebrae

thoracoscopy—New technique that allows surgeons to access the thoracic spine from the side through the chest wall

trigger finger—Form of tenosynovitis; sheath around the tendon in the affected finger becomes irritated and eventually prohibits movement, causing the finger to become locked in a bent position

ultrasound—Medical imaging technique that produces high-frequency sound waves and bounces those waves off of tissues in the body; also known as sonograms

vasodilation—Condition where blood vessels widen in response to the release of prostaglandins when a tendon or ligament is injured to increase blood flow to the uninjured area and thus begin the healing process

whiplash—Range of injuries to the neck caused by or related to a sudden distortion of the neck

X-ray—Medical imaging technique that takes images of the bones and other hard tissues in the body

References

Barnes, Patricia M., and Barbara Bloom. 2008. *National Health Statistics Reports*, no. 12 (December 12, 2008): National Center for Health Statistics. Available from www.nccam.nih.gov/news/2008/nhsr12.pdf.

Benjamin, Ben E. 1984. *Listen to Your Pain: The Active Person's Guide to Understanding, Identifying, and Treating Pain and Injury.* New York: Penguin Books.

Benjamin, Ben E. 2006. Essential skills: Massage in an orthopedic context—Correcting common misperceptions about pain and injury. *Massage & Bodywork*, August/September.

Boden, S.D., D.O. Davis, T.S. Dina, N.J. Patronas, and S.W. Wiesel. 1990. Abnormal magnetic-resonance scans of the lumbar spine in asymptomatic subjects: A prospective investigation. *Journal of Bone and Joint Surgery* 72 (3): 403–408.

Borenstein, D.G., J.W. O'Mara Jr, S.D. Boden, W.C. Lauerman, A. Jacobson, C. Platenberg, D. Schellinger, and S.W. Wiesel. 2001. The value of magnetic resonance imaging of the lumbar spine to predict low-back pain in asymptomatic subjects. *Journal of Bone and Joint Surgery* 83-A (9): 1306–1311.

Crane, David, and Peter A.M. Everts. 2008. Platelet rich plasma (PRP) matrix grafts. *Practical Pain Management*, January/February: 12–26.

Dagenais, S., O. Oqunseitan, S. Haldeman, S. Wooley, J.R. Wooley, and R.L. Newcomb. 2006. Side effects and adverse events related to intraligamentous injection of sclerosing solutions (prolotherapy) for back and neck pain: A survey of practitioners. *Archives of Physical Medicine and Rehabilitation* 87 (July): 909–913.

Devor, Marshall. 2006. Centralization, central sensitization, and neuropathic pain: Focus on "Sciatic chronic constriction injury produces cell-type-specific changes in the electrophysiological properties of rat substantia gelatinosa neurons." *Journal of Neurophysiology* 96: 522–523. Available from http://jn.physiology.org/cgi/content/full/96/2/522.

Dommerholt, Jan, Orlando Mayoral del Moral, and Christian Grobli. 2006. Trigger point dry needling. *Journal of Manual and Manipulative Therapy* 14 (4:) E70–E87.

Dorman, T. and R.G. Klein. 1991. Treatment for spinal pain arising in ligaments using prolotherapy: A retrospective study. *Journal of Orthopedic Medicine* 13 (1): 13–19.

Ducharme J., and C. Barber. 1995. A prospective blinded study on emergency pain assessment and therapy. *Journal of Emergency Medicine* 13: 571–575.

Edwards, S., and J. Calandruccio. 2003. Autologous blood injections for refractory lateral epicondylitis. *The Journal of Hand Surgery* 28 (2): 272–278.

Faber, William J., and Morton Walker. 2007. *Pain, Pain, Go Away*. Charleston, SC: BookSurge Publishing.

Galm, R., M. Frohling, M. Rittmeister, and E. Schmitt. 1998. Sacroiliac joint dysfunction in patients with imaging-proven lumbar disc herniation. *European Spine Journal* 7 (6): 450–453.

Groopman, Jerome. 2008. *How Doctors Think*. Boston, MA: Houghton Mifflin.

Guru, V., and I. Dubinsky. 2000. The patient vs. caregiver perception of acute pain in the emergency department. *Journal of Emergency Medicine*, no. 18: 7–12.

Gwynne, S.C. 2005. Dr. Evil. *Texas Monthly*. September.

Hanley, Edward N., Jr. 1992. The cost of surgical intervention for lumbar disc herniation. In *Clinical Efficacy and Outcome in the Diagnosis and Treatment of Low Back Pain*, edited by James N. Weinstein, American Academy of Orthopaedic Surgery. New York: Raven Press.

Hauser, Ross A., and Marion A. Hauser. 2004. *Prolo Your Pain Away: Curing Chronic Pain with Prolotherapy*. 2nd ed. Oak Park, IL: Beulah Land Press.

Heck, R.K., A.M. O'Malley, E.L. Kellum, T.B. Donovan, A. Elizey, and D.A. Witte. 2007. Errors in the MRI evaluation of musculoskeletal tumors and tumorlike lesions. *Clinical Orthopaedics and Related Research*, no. 459 (June): 28–33.

Herper, M., and R. Langrett. 2006. Dangerous devices. *Forbes*, November 27.

Hotze, S. F. 2007. *Hormones, Health, and Happiness*. Houston, TX: Forrest Publishing.

Jensen, M.C., M.N. Brant-Zawadzki, N. Obuchowski, M.T. Modic, D. Malkasian, and J.S. Ross. 1994. Magnetic resonance imaging of the lumbar spine in people without back pain. *New England Journal of Medicine* 331 (2): 69–73.

Johnston, C.C., A.J. Gagnon, L. Fullerton, C. Common, M. Ladores, and S. Forlini. 1998. One-week survey of pain intensity on admission to and discharge from the emergency department: A pilot study. *Journal of Emergency Medicine* 16: 377–382.

Khan, K.M., J.L. Cook, P. Kannus, N. Maffulli, and S.F. Bonar. 2002. Time to abandon the tendinitis myth: Painful, overuse tendon conditions have a non-inflammatory pathology. *British Medical Journal*, 16 (March): 626–627.

Kim, L.S., L.J. Axelrod, P. Howard, N. Buratovich, and R.F. Waters. 2006. Efficacy of methylsulfonylmethane (MSM) in osteoarthritis pain of the knee: a pilot clinical trial. *Osteoarthritis and Cartilage* 14 (3): 286–294.

Kusunose, Randall. 1992. Strain and counterstrain. In *Rational Manual Therapies*, John V. Basmajian and Richard E. Nyberg. Baltimore, MD: Williams & Wilkins.

Linetsky, F., et al. In press. Regenerative injection therapy. In *Interventional Techniques in Chronic Non-Spinal Pain*. Paducah, KY: ASIPP Publishing.

Liu, Y. 1983. An in situ study of the influence of schlerosing solution in a rabbit medial collateral ligament and its junction strength. *Connective Tissue Research* 2: 95–102.

Maetzel A., and L. Li. 2002. The economic burden of low back pain: A review of studies published between 1996–2001. *Best Practice and Research Clinical Rheumatology* 16 (1): 23–30.

Maynard, J. 1985. Morphological and biomechanical effects of sodium morrhuate on tendons. *Journal of Orthopedic Research* 3: 236–248.

Mozes, A. 2008. New twist on treatment of foot pain. *U.S. News and World Report*. December.

National Center for Health Statistics. 2006. NCHS data on injuries [injury factsheet], June 30, 2006. Available from http://www.cdc.gov/nchs/data/factsheets/injury.pdf.

National Institute of Neurological Disorders and Stroke. Carpal tunnel syndrome [fact sheet]. National Institutes of Health. Available from www.ninds.nih.gov/disorders/carpal_tunnel/detail_carpal_tunnel.htm.

Pai S., L.J. Sundaram. 2004. Low back pain: An economic assessment in the United States. *Orthopedic Clinics of North America*, no. 35: 1–5.

Passik, S.D., K.L. Kirsh, L. Whitcomb, R.K. Portenoy, N.P. Katz, L. Kleinman, S.L. Dodd, and J.R. Schein. 2004. A new tool to assess and document pain outcomes in chronic pain patients receiving opioid therapy. *Clinical Therapeutics*, no. 26: 552–561.

Petrack, E.M., N.C. Christopher, and J. Kriwinsky. 1997. Pain management in the emergency department: Patterns of analgesic utilization. *Pediatrics*, no. 99: 71–74.

Pisetsky, D.S., and S. Flamholtz Trien. 1992. *The Duke University Medical Center Book of Arthritis*. New York, NY: Fawcett Columbine.

Reeves, K.D., and K. Hassanein. 2000. Randomized prospective double-blind placebo-controlled study of dextrose prolotherapy for knee osteoarthritis with or without ACL laxity. *Alternative Therapies* 6 (2): 68–80.

Sobel, D., and A.C. Klein. 1989. *Arthritis: What Worked*. New York: St. Martin's Press.

Theodosakis, J. 2003. *Arthritis Cure*. New York: St. Martin's Press.

Tindel, Nathaniel L., and Tamar Haspel. 2007. *I've Got Your Back: The Truth About Spine Surgery Straight from a Surgeon*. New York: New American Library.

Todd, K.H., E.P. Sloan, C. Chen, S. Eder, and K. Wamstad. 2002. Survey of pain etiology, management practices, and patient satisfaction in two urban emergency departments. *Canadian Journal of Emergency Medical Care*, no. 4: 252–256.

Todd, K.H., J. Ducharme, M. Choiniere, C.S. Crandall, D.E. Fosnocht, P. Homel, P. Tanabe, and PEMI Study Group. 2007. Pain in the emergency department: Results of the pain and emergency medicine initiative (PEMI) multicenter study. *Journal of Pain*, no. 8: 460–466.

U.S. Department of Labor. 2007. *Nonfatal Occupational Injuries and Illnesses Requiring Days away from Work, 2007*. Bureau of Labor Statistics. Available from http://www.bls.gov/news.release/pdf/osh2.pdf.

Weishaupt, D., M. Zanetti, J. Hodler, and N. Boos. 1998. MR imaging of the lumbar spine: Prevalence of intervertebral disc extrusion and sequestration, nerve root compression, end plate abnormalities, and osteoarthritis of the facet joints in asymptomatic volunteers. *Radiology* 209 (3): 661–666.

Yelland, M.J., P.P. Glasziou, N. Bogduk, P.J. Schluter, and M. McKernon. 2004. Prolotherapy injections, saline injections, and exercise for low back pain: A randomized study. *Spine*, 29 (1): 9–16.

Zucherman, James, and Jerome Schofferman. Pathology of failed back surgical syndrome: The lesions that cause the pain. Spinedr. Available from www.spine-dr.com/site/surgery/surgery_article2.html.

Acknowledgments

I want to thank God, from whom all good things come. Hopefully, the information in this book will be the answer to the prayers of some readers. I wish to honor my father for his inspiration and support. To my children, Alec, Chris, Danielle, Matt, and Anna — I hope I can be an inspiration and support for you. Thanks to Ben Cowart for giving me that last little push to follow what I was meant to do. Thanks to Sandra Paton for her help in writing the book. Of course the staff at Greanleaf Book Group was invaluable, particularly Lari Bishop, Alan Grimes, and Justin Branch.

To my staff Elva, Maggie, and Blanca, thanks for being like family and helping me through all the challenges of a practice and busy life. Thanks to Joanne for all the good years together.

With healthcare costs becoming excessive and unaffordable, the nonsurgical options outlined in this book will help demonstrate that the most expensive care is not always the best care. I want to acknowledge the inspiration that Dr. Jason Theodosakis, author of *The Arthritis Cure*, and Dr. Steven F. Hotze, author of *Hormones, Health, and Happiness*, provided in their books, making me realize that not all the best medicine is learned in medical schools or provided by pharmaceutical companies.

Index